CLINICAL APPLICATION OF MECHANICAL VENTILATION

WORKBOOK

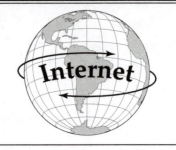
A Division of Thomson Learning™

CLINICAL APPLICATION OF MECHANICAL VENTILATION

WORKBOOK

SECOND EDITION

David W. Chang, Ed.D., R.R.T.
Director of Clinical Education
Respiratory Therapy
Athens Technical College
Athens, Georgia

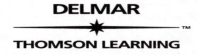

DELMAR

THOMSON LEARNING

Africa • Australia • Canada • Denmark • Japan • Mexico • New Zealand • Philippines
Puerto Rico • Singapore • Spain • United Kingdom • United States

NOTICE TO THE READER

Publisher does not warrant or guarantee any of the products described herein or perform any independent analysis in connection with any of the product information contained herein. Publisher does not assume, and expressly disclaims, any obligation to obtain and include information other than that provided to it by the manufacturer.

The reader is expressly warned to consider and adopt all safety precautions that might be indicated by the activities described herein and to avoid all potential hazards. By following the instructions contained herein, the reader willingly assumes all risks in connection with such instructions.

The Publisher makes no representation or warranties of any kind, including but not limited to, the warranties of fitness for particular purpose or merchantability, nor are any such representations implied with respect to the material set forth herein, and the publisher takes no responsibility with respect to such material. The publisher shall not be liable for any special, consequential, or exemplary damages resulting, in whole or in part, from the readers' use of, or reliance upon, this material.

CPT five-digit codes, nomenclature, and other data are copyright © 1999 American Medical Association. All rights reserved. No fee schedules, basic unit, relative values, or related listings are included in CPT. The AMA assumes no liability for the data contained herein.

Delmar Staff:

Health Care Publishing Director: William Brottmiller

Acquisitions Editor: Candice Janco

Developmental Editor: Deb Flis

Art/Design Coordinator: Rich Killar

Executive Marketing Manager: Dawn F. Gerrain

Marketing Coordinator: Nina Lontrato

For more information, contact Delmar, 3 Columbia Circle, PO Box 15015, Albany, NY 12212–0515; or find us on the World Wide Web at http://www.delmar.com

Asia
Thomson Learning
60 Albert Street, #15-01
Albert Complex
Singapore 189969
Tel: 65 336 6411
Fax: 65 336 7411

Japan
Thomson Learning
Palaceside Building 5F
1-1-1 Hitotsubashi, Chiyoda-ku
Tokyo 100 0003 Japan
Tel: 813 5218 6544
Fax: 813 5218 6551

Australia/New Zealand
Nelson/Thomson Learning
102 Dodds Street
South Melbourne, Victoria 3205
Australia
Tel: 61 39 685 4111
Fax: 61 39 685 4199

UK/Europe/Middle East
Thomson Learning
Berkshire House
168–173 High Holborn
London
WC1V7AA United Kingdom
Tel: 44 171 497 1422
Fax: 44 171 497 1426

Thomas Nelson & Sons LTD
Nelson House
Mayfield Road
Walton-on-Thames
KT 12 5PL United Kingdom
Tel: 44 1932 2522111
Fax: 44 1932 246574

Latin America
Thomson Learning
Seneca, 53
Colonia Polanco
11560 Mexico D.F. Mexico
Tel: 525-281-2906
Fax: 525-281-2656

South Africa
Thomson Learning
Zonnebloem Building
Constantia Square
526 Sixteenth Road
P.O. Box 2459
Halfway House, 1685
South Africa
Tel: 27 11 805 4819
Fax: 27 11 805 3648

Canada
Nelson/Thomson Learning
1120 Birchmount Road
Scarborough, Ontario
Canada M1K 5G4
Tel: 416-752-9100
Fax: 416-752-8102

Spain
Thomson Learning
Calle Magallanes, 25
28015-MADRID
ESPANA
Tel: 34 91 446 33 50
Fax: 34 91 445 62 18

International Headquarters
Thomson Learning
International Division
290 Harbor Drive, 2nd Floor
Stamford, CT 06902-7477
Tel: 203-969-8700
Fax: 203-969-8751

Library of Congress Cataloging-in-Publication Data

ISBN 0-7668-1377-0

CONTENTS

CHAPTER ONE

PRINCIPLES OF MECHANICAL VENTILATION

INTRODUCTION

1. The general purpose of mechanical ventilation includes all of the following *except*:
   A. correction of hypoxemia.
   B. elimination of carbon dioxide.
   C. support of ventilatory failure.
   D. compensation of acid-base imbalance.

2. Mechanical ventilation is usually NOT indicated in conditions such as:
   A. ventilatory failure.
   B. metabolic acidosis.
   C. chest trauma.
   D. post-operative recovery.

3. One of the most frequent uses of mechanical ventilation is for the management of _____ (preoperative, postoperative) patients _____ (before receiving, recovering from) anesthesia and medications.

4. Complete the six pathophysiological factors or changes below that may lead to the use of mechanical ventilation.
   (1) _____ (High, Low) airway resistance
   (2) _____ (High, Low) lung compliance
   (3) _____ (Hyperventilation, Hypoventilation)
   (4) _____ (Hyperoxia, V/Q mismatch)
   (5) _____ (Intrapulmonary, Systemic) shunting
   (6) _____ (Anemia, Diffusion defect)

5. Patients who require mechanical ventilation usually have developed ventilatory failure, oxygenation failure, or both.

   (TRUE/FALSE)

AIRWAY RESISTANCE

6. Airway resistance is the degree of _____ obstruction in the airways.

7. Describe the factors affecting the airway resistance during mechanical ventilation.

   _____

8. Air flow obstruction may be caused by all of the following changes *except*:
   A. increased lung compliance.
   B. retained secretions in the airways.
   C. neoplasm of the bronchial muscle structure.
   D. tumors compressing the airway.

9. When the radius of an airway decreases by _____ (25%, 50%, 75%, 160%) of its original size, the driving pressure needed to maintain the same air flow must increase by a factor of _____ (2-fold, 16-fold, 100-fold).

10 to 12. Match the type of air flow obstruction with the clinical conditions that may increase a patient's airway resistance.

TYPE	CLINICAL CONDITIONS
10. COPD	A. Condensation in ventilator circuit
11. Mechanical obstruction	B. Epiglottitis
12. Infection	C. Chronic asthma

13. During mechancial ventilation, one of the strategies to reduce the air flow resistance is to:
   A. lengthen the endotracheal tube.
   B. use the smallest endotracheal tube possible.
   C. remove the secretions in the endotracheal tube.
   D. add water to the ventilator circuit.

14. Airway resistance and work of breathing are _____ (directly, inversely) related. In other words, the work of breathing is _____ (increased, decreased) in conditions of high airway resistance.

15. If the work of breathing cannot keep pace with the increase of airway resistance, the air flow will _____ (increase, decrease).

16. In order to overcome air flow resistance, patients with chronic airway obstruction typically use a breathing pattern that is _____ (deep and slow, shallow and fast).

17. Under respiratory stress or hypoxia, patients with restrictive lung disease breathe _____ (deep and slow, shallow and fast) since air flow resistance _____ (is, is not) the primary disturbance in these patients.

18. When an abnormally high airway resistance is sustained over a long time, all of the following may occur with the *exception* of:
   A. fatigue of the respiratory muscles.
   B. metabolic alkalosis.
   C. ventilatory failure.
   D. oxygenation failure.

LUNG COMPLIANCE

19. Given: Corrected V_T = 600 mL, Peak airway pressure = 45 cm H_2O, Plateau pressure = 35 cm H_2O, PEEP = 5 cm H_2O. Calculate the static compliance (C_{ST}) and dynamic compliance (C_{DYN}).
    A. C_{ST} = 13 mL/cm H_2O, C_{DYN} = 17 mL/cm H_2O
    B. C_{ST} = 15 mL/cm H_2O, C_{DYN} = 20 mL/cm H_2O
    C. C_{ST} = 17 mL/cm H_2O, C_{DYN} = 13 mL/cm H_2O
    D. C_{ST} = 20 mL/cm H_2O, C_{DYN} = 15 mL/cm H_2O

20. Given: Corrected V_T = 660 mL, Peak airway pressure = 60 cm H_2O, Plateau pressure = 40 cm H_2O, PEEP = 10 cm H_2O. Calculate the static compliance (C_{ST}) and dynamic compliance (C_{DYN}).
    A. C_{ST} = 11 mL/cm H_2O, C_{DYN} = 17 mL/cm H_2O
    B. C_{ST} = 13 mL/cm H_2O, C_{DYN} = 22 mL/cm H_2O
    C. C_{ST} = 17 mL/cm H_2O, C_{DYN} = 11 mL/cm H_2O
    D. C_{ST} = 22 mL/cm H_2O, C_{DYN} = 13 mL/cm H_2O

21. Since the peak airway pressure is _____ (equal to, higher than, lower than) the plateau pressure, which of the following statements is true concerning the calculated compliance values?
    A. The dynamic compliance is same as the static compliance.
    B. The dynamic compliance is greater than the static compliance.
    C. The dynamic compliance is lower than the static compliance.
    D. The dynamic and static compliance values are usually greater than 35 mL/cm H_2O.

22. _____ (High, Low) compliance makes lung expansion difficult whereas _____ (high, low) compliance leads to poor elastic recoil of the lung tissues, incomplete exhalation, and CO_2 retention.

23. _____ (High, Low) compliance or _____ (high, low) elastance means that the volume change is small per unit pressure change. Under this condition, the lungs are considered "stiff" or _____ (compliant, non-compliant).

24. Compliance and work of breathing are _____ (directly, inversely) related. In other words, the work of breathing is _____ (increased, decreased) in conditions of *low* compliance.

25. If the work of breathing cannot keep pace with the decrease of compliance, the lung volume will _____ (increase, decrease) as a result.

26. When an abnormally *low* compliance is sustained over a long time, all of the following may occur with the exception of:
    A. oxygenation failure.
    B. ventilatory failure.
    C. respiratory muscle fatigue.
    D. renal failure.

27. Mr. Jones, a patient diagnosed with adult respiratory distress syndrome, has a static compliance of 15 mL/cm H_2O (*normal is 40 to 60 mL/cm H_2O*). Based on the compliance value, which of the following assumptions is most reliable?

A. The patient's functional residual capacity is increased.

B. The elastic recoil of the lungs is decreased.

C. The patient may have an obstructive lung defect.

D. The patient's work of breathing is increased.

28. When the compliance value is extremely high as seen in patients with emphysema, exhalation is often _____ (improved, incomplete) due to a(n) _____ (increase, decrease) of lung elasticity.

29. High compliance measurement is usually related to conditions of _____ (elevated, decreased) functional residual capacity, _____ (obstructive, restrictive) lung defect, air flow obstruction, incomplete exhalation, and poor gas exchange.

30. In general, the static compliance is affected by changes in the _____ (airway, lung parenchyma). An example for this condition is _____ (bronchospasm, pneumonia, main bronchus intubation).

31. Airway obstruction primarily leads to changes in the _____ (static, dynamic) compliance.

32. Since static compliance is measured when there is _____ (high, little or no) air flow, airway resistance _____ (is, is not) a determining factor of the static compliance measurement.

33. Static compliance reflects the _____ (elastic, non-elastic) properties of the lung and chest wall and it is known as the _____ (elastic, non-elastic) resistance.

34. Since dynamic compliance is measured when air flow is _____ (present, absent), airway resistance _____ (is, is not) a determining factor of the compliance measurement.

35. Dynamic compliance reflects the condition of the:
    A. airway resistance (non-elastic resistance).
    B. elastic properties of the lung and chest wall (elastic resistance).
    C. A and B.

36. In general, conditions causing changes in the static compliance invoke _____ (similar, different) changes in the dynamic compliance. For example, atelectasis _____ (increases, decreases) the _____ (static, dynamic, static and dynamic) compliance measurement.

37. In conditions where the airway resistance is increased, the _____ (static, dynamic) compliance changes independently without a corresponding change of the _____ (static, dynamic) compliance. For example, bronchospasm _____ (increases, decreases) the _____ (static, dynamic) compliance only.

38. In non-intubated subjects, the normal dynamic compliance is between _____ and _____ mL/cm H_2O and the normal static compliance is between _____ and _____ mL/cm H_2O).

DEADSPACE VENTILATION

39. Deadspace ventilation is defined as wasted ventilation or a condition in which _____ (ventilation, pulmonary blood flow) is in excess of _____ (ventilation, pulmonary blood flow).

40. The anatomic deadspace of a 140-lb patient may be estimated to be _____ (70, 100, 140, 180) mL.

41. Decrease in tidal volume causes a relatively _____ (higher, lower) anatomic deadspace to tidal volume (V_D/V_T) ratio.

42. Alveolar deadspace ventilation occurs when the ventilated alveoli are _____ (overly, not adequately) perfused by the pulmonary circulation.

43. Alveolar deadspace ventilation may be caused by all of the following conditions *except*:
    A. pulmonary vasoconstriction.
    B. congestive heart failure.
    C. blood loss.
    D. atelectasis.

44. Physiologic deadspace is the _____ (sum, difference, product) of anatomic and alveolar deadspace volumes. Under normal conditions, the physiologic deadspace is about the same as the _____ (anatomic, alveolar) deadspace.

45. Measurement of the physiologic deadspace to tidal volume ratio (V_D/V_T) requires a(n):
    A. arterial blood sample.
    B. mixed expired gas sample.
    C. pulmonary artery blood sample.
    D. A and B.

46. The physiologic deadspace to tidal volume ratio (V_D/V_T) is calculated by:
    A. $V_D/V_T = (PaCO_2 - PECO_2)$.
    B. $V_D/V_T = (PaCO_2 - PECO_2) \times PaCO_2$.
    C. $V_D/V_T = (PaCO_2 - PECO_2) / PaCO_2$.
    D. $V_D/V_T = (PaCO_2 \times PECO_2) / PaCO_2$.

47. V_D/V_T of less than 60% reflects _____ (normal, abnormal) ventilatory function upon successful weaning from mechanical ventilation.

48. Prolonged and excessive deadspace ventilation causes inefficient ventilation, muscle fatigue, ventilatory and oxygenation failure.

    (TRUE/FALSE)

VENTILATORY FAILURE

49. Define ventilatory failure.

_____

_____

50. The key feature of ventilatory failure is _____ (hypercapnia, hypocapnia) or significant _____ (increase, decrease) of arterial PCO$_2$.

51. When carbon dioxide _____ (removal, production) exceeds its _____ (removal, production), respiratory _____ (acidosis, alkalosis) is the end result.

52 to 56. Match the mechanisms leading to the development of ventilatory failure with the typical findings. Use each answer only once.

MECHANISM	CLINICAL FINDING
52. Hypoventilation	A. Q$_S$/Q$_T$ greater than 20% (>30% in critical shunt)
53. Persistent V/Q Mismatch	B. Low barometric pressure as in high altitude
54. Persistent Intrapulmonary Shunt	C. Gas diffusion rate less than 75% of predicted normal
55. Persistent Diffusion Defect	D. PaCO$_2$ greater than 45 mm Hg (>50 to 60 mm Hg for COPD patients)
56. Persistent Reduction of P$_I$O$_2$	E. Hypoxemia that responds well to oxygen therapy

57. Which of the following conditions is *not* likely a cause of alveolar hypoventilation?
    A. metabolic acidosis
    B. depression of breathing centers
    C. neuromuscular disease
    D. airway obstruction

58. In reviewing a patient's chart, the admitting note states that the patient was *hypoventilating* upon arrival at the emergency department. This assessment is based on an increase of the patient's _____ (alveolar ventilation, deadspace ventilation, arterial carbon dioxide tension).

59. Based on the equation: V$_A$ = V$_T$ – V$_D$, a patient's alveolar volume can be increased by:
    A. increasing the tidal volume (V$_T$).
    B. increasing the deadspace volume (V$_D$).
    C. decreasing the tidal volume (V$_T$).
    D. decreasing the tidal volume (V$_T$) and deadspace volume (V$_D$).

60. Since minute ventilation (V$_A$) is a function of the tidal volume (V$_T$), deadspace volume (V$_D$) and respiratory rate (RR) as shown in the equation: (V$_A$) = (V$_T$ – V$_D$) × RR, hypoventilation can be corrected by:
    A. decreasing the V$_T$.
    B. decreasing the RR.
    C. increasing the RR.
    D. increasing the V$_D$.

61. A physician asks you to monitor Mr. Smith's *ventilatory* status, you would measure the patient's _____ (pH, PaO$_2$, PaCO$_2$, respiratory rate) on an as needed basis.

62. Based on the equation: $V_A = VCO_2 / PaCO_2$, an increase of carbon dioxide production (VCO_2) would cause a(n) _____ (increase, decrease) of the arterial carbon dioxide tension ($PaCO_2$) level. (Assume the VA remains unchanged.)

63. Define V/Q mismatch.

_____

64. A _____ (high, low) V/Q ratio may be seen in pulmonary embolism where the pulmonary _____ (ventilation, perfusion) is reduced.

65. In airway obstruction, pulmonary _____ (ventilation, perfusion) is reduced and it leads to a _____ (high, low) V/Q ratio.

66. Hypoxemia caused by uncomplicated V/Q mismatch is generally _____ (readily, not) reversible by oxygen therapy alone.

67. Define intrapulmonary shunting.

_____

68. Define refractory hypoxemia.

_____

69. Since shunted pulmonary blood flow _____ (does, does not) come in contact with ventilated and oxygenated alveoli, oxygen therapy is usually an _____ (effective, ineffective) treatment for shunting.

70. A hemodynamic study reveals that Ms. Jamison's shunt percent is 35%. This may be interpreted as a _____ (normal, mild, significant, critical) intrapulmonary shunt.

71. The *estimated* physiologic shunt equation for a critically ill patient is:
    A. Estimated $Q_S/Q_T = (CcO_2 - CaO_2) / [2 + (CcO_2 - CaO_2)]$.
    B. Estimated $Q_S/Q_T = (CcO_2 - CaO_2) / [3.5 + (CcO_2 - CaO_2)]$.
    C. Estimated $Q_S/Q_T = (CcO_2 - CaO_2) / [5 + (CcO_2 - CaO_2)]$.
    D. Estimated $Q_S/Q_T = (CcO_2 - CaO_2) / [16 + (CcO_2 - CaO_2)]$.

72. As shown below, the *classic* physiologic shunt equation requires _____ (one, two, three) blood sample(s).

    Classic $Q_S/Q_T = (CcO_2 - CaO_2) / (CcO_2 - CvO_2)$

73 to 76. Match the causes of decreased diffusion rate with the clinical conditions. Use each answer only once.

TYPE OF DIFFUSION PROBLEM	CLINICAL CONDITIONS
73. Decrease of pressure gradient	A. Pulmonary edema, retained secretions
74. Thickening of A-c membrane	B. Tachycardia
75. Decreased surface area of A-c membrane	C. Emphysema, pulmonary fibrosis
76. Insufficient time for diffusion	D. High altitude, fire combustion

OXYGENATION FAILURE

77. Oxygenation failure is defined as severe _____ (hyperventilation, hypoventilation, hypoxemia) that does not respond to moderate to high levels of _____ (mechanical ventilation, supplemental oxygen).

78. Arterial PO_2 measures the amount of oxygen _____ (dissolved in the plasma, combined with hemoglobin) and it _____ (does, does not) accurately reflect a patient's overall oxygenation status in:
    A. atelectasis.
    B. chronic airway obstruction.
    C. post-operative recovery.
    D. carbon monoxide inhalation.

79. Differentiate hypoxemia and hypoxia.

80. Hypoxia can occur with a PaO_2 of 85 mm Hg.

    (TRUE/FALSE)

81. The important clinical signs of oxygenation failure and hypoxia include all of the following *except*:
    A. hypothermia.
    B. dyspnea.
    C. tachypnea.
    D. tachycardia.

CLINICAL CONDITIONS LEADING TO MECHANCIAL VENTILATION

82. Depressed respiratory drive is one of the indications for mechanical ventilation. Which of the following conditions is *least* likely to affect a patient's normal respiratory drive?
    A. spinal cord injury at cervical-2 (C-2) level
    B. drug overdose
    C. chest trauma
    D. head injury

83. Excessive ventilatory workload is one of the indications for mechanical ventilation. Which of the following conditions is *least* likely to increase a patient's ventilatory workload?
    A. air flow obstruction
    B. increased deadspace ventilation
    C. acute lung injury
    D. post-anesthesia recovery

84. Failure of the ventilatory pump is one of the indications for mechanical ventilation. Which of the following conditions does *not* normally lead to failure of the ventilatory pump?

A. electrolyte imbalance

B. head injury

C. chest trauma

D. fatigue of respiratory muscles

CHAPTER TWO

EFFECTS OF POSITIVE PRESSURE VENTILATION

PULMONARY CONSIDERATIONS

1. During spontaneous ventilation, the diaphragm and other respiratory muscles create gas flow by _____ (increasing, decreasing) the pleural, alveolar, and airway pressures.

2. When the alveolar and airway pressures _____ (go over, drop below) the atmospheric pressure, air flows into the lungs.

3. In negative pressure ventilation, the pressures in the airways, alveoli, and pleura during inspiration are _____ (increased, decreased) whereas in positive pressure ventilation the same pressures are _____ (increased, decreased).

4. With normal airway resistance and compliance, a higher positive pressure applied to the lungs results in a _____ (larger, smaller) tidal volume.

5. With pressure limited ventilators, when the peak airway pressure is reached prematurely, the tidal volume delivered to the patient will be _____ (higher, lower) than normal.

6. All of the following clinical conditions may cause the inspiratory phase to end prematurely *except*:
   A. circuit disconnect.
   B. airway obstruction.
   C. kinking of endotracheal tube.
   D. low lung compliance.

7. Mechanical ventilators cannot effectively provide ventilation if they are unable to reach the peak airway pressure. This condition may be seen in:
   A. kinking of ventilator circuit.
   B. low lung compliance.
   C. high airway resistance.
   D. endotracheal tube cuff leak.

8. When mechanical ventilation is provided by a pressure-limited ventilator, the _____ (volume, pressure) is preset and the _____ (volume, pressure) delivered by the ventilator is *variable*.

9. When mechanical ventilation is provided by a volume-limited ventilator, the _____ (volume, pressure) is preset and the _____ (volume, pressure) generated by the ventilator is *variable*.

10. In patients with _____ (compliant, noncompliant) lungs, the effects of positive pressure on the cardiac output is less severe because _____ (more, less) pressure is transmitted from the airways to the lung parenchyma.

CARDIOVASCULAR CONSIDERATIONS

11. Positive pressure ventilation typically _____ (increases, decreases) the mean airway pressure (MAWP) and _____ (increases, decreases) a patient's cardiac output.

12. A ventilator patient has a calculated mean airway pressure (MAWP) of 40 cm H_2O and the physician would like to lower it in order to minimize the cardiovascular side effects. You would:

    A. decrease the flow rate ($\uparrow$ I time).

    B. increase the respiratory rate.

    C. decrease the tidal volume ($\downarrow$ peak inspiratory pressure).

    D. increase the positive end-expiratory pressure.

13. Given: O_2 Content $\times$ Cardiac Output = O_2 Delivery

    Since positive pressure ventilation commonly leads to a(n) _____ (increase, decrease) of the cardiac output, the oxygen delivery is likely to be _____ (increased, reduced) as a result. (Assume the oxygen content remains unchanged.)

14. In patients with cardiopulmonary disease or compromised cardiovascular reserve, positive pressure ventilation may cause the blood pressure measurements to _____ (increase, decrease).

15. Due to the thoracic pump mechanism, an increase of tidal volume causes a decrease of venous return to the left ventricle in _____ (hypertensive, hypotensive) patients.

16. In hypertensive patients, use of a large tidal volume _____ (increases, decrease) venous return to the left ventricle due to the thoracic pump mechanism.

17. During mechanical ventilation, the thoracic pump mechanism _____ (facilitates, restricts) the outflow of blood from the right ventricle. For this reason, high positive pressure and large tidal volume have been used in children with right ventricular dysfunction to _____ (increase, reduce) the work load of the right heart.

HEMODYNAMIC CONSIDERATIONS

18. Positive pressure ventilation causes a(n) _____ (increase, decrease) of the intrathoracic pressure and compression of the pulmonary blood vessels. This condition causes an overall _____ (increase, decrease) in ventricular output, stroke volume, and pressure readings.

19. The degree of severity of hemodynamic changes is NOT related to the level of airway pressures, lung volume, and compliance characteristics of the patient.

    (TRUE/FALSE)

20. The intrathoracic pressure is _____ (increased, decreased) during mechanical ventilation because the positive pressure applied to the lungs causes _____ (expansion, compression) of the lung parenchyma against the chest wall.

21. During the *inspiratory* phase of positive pressure ventilation, a fraction of the _____ (systemic, pulmonary) blood volume is shifted to the _____ (systemic, pulmonary) circulation. This causes a transient _____ (increase, decrease) of the pulmonary blood volume.

22. A higher intrathoracic pressure _____ (enhances, impedes) the systemic blood return to the right ventricle. This results in a _____ (higher, lower) venous return and a higher central venous pressure (CVP) reading.

23. A lower venous return to the right ventricle leads to a _____ (higher, lower) right ventricular output and a _____ (higher, lower) blood volume in the pulmonary arterial system.

24. Since volume and pressure are _____ (directly, inversely) related, a lower blood volume in the pulmonary arterial system leads to a _____ (higher, lower) pulmonary arterial pressure (PAP) reading.

25. As the left ventricle receives less blood from the pulmonary circulation, the left ventricular output is _____ (increased, unchanged, decreased).

26. In the absence of compensation by increasing the heart rate, decrease of right and left ventricular stroke volumes generally leads to a decreased cardiac output.

    (TRUE/FALSE)

27. The hemodynamic effects of PEEP are highly variable and dependent on a patient's condition. In general, PEEP causes a(n) _____ (increase, decrease) of the pulmonary artery pressure and the central venous pressure but a(n) _____ (increase, decrease) of the aortic pressure and cardiac output.

28. PEEP leads to a(n) _____ (increase, decrease) of the pulmonary artery pressure (PAP) because PEEP causes significant compression of the pulmonary blood vessels.

29. Increase of PAP causes a higher right ventricular pressure and hinders the blood return from systemic circulation to right heart. This causes backup of blood flow and a(n) _____ (increase, decrease) of pressure in the systemic venous circulation (i.e., central venous pressure).

30. PEEP leads to a(n) _____ (increase, decrease) of the aortic pressure because of a significant increase of the intrathoracic pressure and significant reduction of the left and right ventricular stroke volumes.

31. PEEP _____ (increases, decreases) the cardiac output for the same reasons leading to a decreased aortic pressure.

RENAL CONSIDERATIONS

32. Besides elimination of wastes and clearance of certain drugs, kidneys are efficient in the regulation of all of the following *except*:
    A. spinal fluid pressure.
    B. fluid balance.

C. electrolyte balance.

D. acid-base balance.

33. The kidneys are highly vascular and at any one time receive about _____ (1%, 5%, 25%, 50%) of the body's circulating blood volume. For this reason, they are highly vulnerable to the decrease of blood flow during positive pressure ventilation.

34. When renal perfusion is decreased, filtration and reabsorption become _____ (more, less) effective. As a result, the urine output is _____ (increased, decreased) as the kidneys try to correct this _____ (hypervolemic, hypovolemic) condition by _____ (releasing, retaining) fluid.

35. For adequate removal of body wastes, the urine output must be above _____ (100 ml, 200 ml, 300 ml, 400 ml) in a 24-hour period. Therefore, a(n) _____ (increased, decreased) urine output is an early sign of renal failure.

36. Inadequate urine output is called _____ and is defined as a urine output of less than _____ ml in 24 hours or less than _____ ml in 8 hours.

37. Other early signs of renal failure include _____ (elevation, reduction) of the serum blood urea nitrogen level to _____ (more than, less than) 20 mg/dl and the creatinine level to _____ (more than, less than) 1.5 mg/dl.

38. During positive presure ventilation, hypoperfusion of the kidneys may _____ (increase, decrease) the rate of drug clearance and lead to a _____ (higher, lower) drug concentration in the circulation.

39. The drug concentration in the circulation may be increased in all of the following renal conditions with the *exception* of:

A. decrease of glomerular filtration rate.

B. decrease of tubular secretion.

C. increase of renal perfusion.

D. decrease of drug reabsorption rate.

HEPATIC CONSIDERATIONS

40. The liver is perfused by about 15% of the total cardiac output and this perfusion rate may be reduced when _____ (oxygen, pressure support, PEEP) is added to positive pressure ventilation.

41. All of the following laboratory measurements may indicate the presence of liver dysfunction with the *exception* of:

A. prothrombin time > 4 seconds over control.

B. pH > 7.50.

C. bilirubin level ≥ 50 mg/L.

D. albumin level ≤ 20 g/L.

42. Clearance of lidocaine, meperidine, propranolol, and verapamil relies on adequate liver function and perfusion. When the hepatic perfusion is inadequate, use of these drugs may lead to a relatively _____ (higher, lower) drug concentration due to _____ (enhanced, impaired) drug clearance.

ABDOMINAL CONSIDERATIONS

43. Increased intra-abdominal pressure (IAP) may transmit the excessive pressure across the diaphragm to the heart and great vessels. In turn, this leads to _____ (increased, decreased) cardiac output, _____ (increased, decreased) renal perfusion, and _____ (increased, decreased) functional residual capacity.

44. Use of PEEP at a level greater than _____ (5, 10, 15) cm H_2O in the presence of high IAP (>20 mmHg) requires caution because of the potentiation of the pressures exerted on the heart and great vessels.

45. Excessive PEEP and IAP _____ (increases, decreases) the functional residual capacity and leads to all of the following complications *except*:
    A. increased atelectasis.
    B. impaired gas exchange.
    C. increased V/Q mismatch.
    D. decreased venous admixture.

NUTRITIONAL CONSIDERATIONS

46. Nutritional balance is vital in the management of critically ill patients as malnutrition may cause _____ (excessive CO_2 production, muscle fatigue) whereas excessive nutritional support may cause _____ (excessive CO_2 production, muscle fatigue).

47. COPD patients have higher caloric needs because of the increased work of breathing associated with chronic air flow obstruction.

    (TRUE/FALSE)

48. Fatigue of the respiratory muscles and ventilatory failure are most likely to occur in conditions where the:
    A. airway resistance is low.
    B. chest wall compliance is high.
    C. lung compliance is low.
    D. work of breathing is low.

49. Besides malnutrition, list four other conditions that may lead to respiratory muscle fatigue.

    _____

    _____

50. Describe the process of undernutrition leading to a reduction of ventilatory efficiency.

    _____

    _____

    _____

51. Inspiratory strengths and endurance may be improved by keeping the daily caloric intake under 400 kcal.

    (TRUE/ FALSE)

52. _____ (More, Less) nutritional supplement is needed for ventilator patients who are hypermetabolic or hypercatabolic due to conditions such as infection, trauma, and burns.

53. For patients with CO_2 retention, a _____ (fat-based, glucose-based) parenteral diet supplement is preferred becasue it provides _____ (more, less) kcal per gram and _____ (higher, lower) CO_2 production.

NEUROLOGICAL CONSIDERATIONS

54. In mechanical ventilation, intentional hyperventilation is sometimes used to reduce the _____ (pH, intrapulmonary pressure, intracranial pressure) in patients with head injury.

55. Sustained hyperventilation of less than 24 hours causes respiratory _____ (acidosis, alkalosis), and a(n) _____ (increase, reduction) of cerebral blood flow and intracranial pressure.

56. List three side effects of prolonged (>24 hours) hyperventilation.

    _____

    _____

57. Hypoventilation and abnormalities in gas exchange can cause all of the following conditions *except*:
    A. hypocapnia.
    B. respiratory acidosis.
    C. hypoxemia.
    D. secondary polycythemia.

58. Mr. Kingston, a patient who was weaned from mechanical ventilation two days ago, complains of pressure headache, motor disturbances, and ocular abnormalities. While talking with him, he appears to have moderate deterioration in his mental status. These complaints and observation are suggestive of:
    A. sustained hyperventilation.
    B. neurological impairment.
    C. electrolyte imbalance.
    D. oxygen toxicity.

59. _____ (Hypercapnia, Hypocapnia) may cause muscle tremor and ocular abnormalities.

60. Muscle tremor is the result of excessive _____ (stimulation, suppression) of the sympathetic nervous system and catecholamine release from the adrenal medulla.

61. Ocular abnormalities are the result of cerebral _____ (vasodilation, vasoconstriction) and _____ (elevation, depression) of intracranial pressure.

62 to 64. Match the pulmonary conditions with the physiologic changes. Use each answer only once.

CONDITION	PHYSIOLOGIC CHANGES
62. Hypercapnia (with normal pH)	A. Impaired cerebral metabolism
63. Hypoxemia	B. Increased cerebral blood flow and intracranial pressure
64. Hypercapnia (with low pH)	C. Decreased mental and motor functions

CHAPTER THREE

CLASSIFICATION OF MECHANICAL VENTILATORS

VENTILATOR CLASSIFICATION

1. A classification system for ventilators is used to learn the _____ (waveform, operational, pressure) characteristics of each ventilator.

2. Ventilators may be classified by their
   A. similarities.
   B. differences.
   C. manufacturers.
   D. A and B only.

VENTILATORY WORK

3. Mechanical ventilators generate gas flow and lung volume by creating a trans-airway _____ (compliance, volume, pressure) gradient.

4. The work of breathing that the patient or ventilator must perform is _____ (directly, inversely) proportional to the pressure required to generate any tidal volume.

5. In order to create sufficient gas flow and adequate lung volume, the patient or ventilator must overcome the opposing force of
   A. compliance.
   B. resistance.
   C. conductance.
   D. A and B only.

6. Change in volume divided by change in pressure equals to the _____ (compliance, resistance, elastance, conductance) measurement.

7. Pressure divided by flow represents the _____ (conductance, compliance, resistance, elastance) measurement.

INPUT POWER

8. Pneumatically powered ventilators use _____ as an energy source for their operation.

9. Give at least two examples of pneumatically powered ventilators.

   _____

10. Electrically powered ventilators may use 120 v 60 Hz alternating current (AC) or 12 v direct current (DC) for a power source. The _____ (AC, DC) is one available in the homes, whereas _____ (AC, DC) is one provided by the batteries.

11. Give at least two examples of electrically powered ventilators.

    _____

12. Name two ventilators that are powered by a combination of pneumatic and electric power sources.

    _____

DRIVE MECHANISM

13. The drive mechanism is the system used by a ventilator to convert the input power to gas flow and tidal volume.

    (TRUE/FALSE)

14. Name the four types of drive mechanisms that may be used on ventilators.

    _____

15. Rotary or linear driven pistons are used to generate _____ (pressure, volume, temperature) to operate a ventilator.

16. Bellows drive ventilators use a bellows to _____ (send, filter, compress) the gas for delivery to the patient.

17. Reducing valve drive ventilators use a reducing valve to create a _____ (volume, pressure, compliance) gradient for delivery of volume.

18. The Bennett PR-2 is a simple ventilator that uses a _____ (piston, bellows, reducing valve) as its drive mechanism.

19. When a ventilator uses microprocessors to open and close the solenoid valves, the process is called a microprocessor controlled _____ (piston, bellows, pressure, pneumatic) drive mechanism.

CONTROL CIRCUIT

20. The control circuit is the system that governs or controls the ventilator _____ or output control valve.

21. An open loop control circuit is one where the desired output is selected and the ventilator achieves the desired output _____ (with additional, without any further) input from the clinician or the ventilator.

22. A closed loop control circuit is one where the _____ (input, output) is constantly adjusted to match the desired _____ (input, output). This type of control circuit may also be referred to as _____ controlled.

23. _____ (Mechanical, Pneumatic, Fluidic, Electric, Electronic) control circuits employ simple machines such as levers, pulleys, or cams to control the drive mechanism.

24. _____ (Mechanical, Pneumatic, Fluidic, Electric, Electronic) control circuits use devices such as valves, nozzles, ducted ejectors, and diaphragms.

25. Fluidic control circuits operate on the principle of the _____ (Fluidic, Halo, Coanda) Effect by using gas flow and pressure to control the ventilator functions.

26. Electric control circuits utilize simple electrical _____ (sensors, breakers, switches) to control the drive mechanism.

27. _____ control circuits use resistors, diodes, transistors, integrated circuits and sometimes microprocessors to control the drive mechanisms of the ventilators.

CONTROL VARIABLES

28. Name the four control variables that may be found on mechanical ventilators.

_____

29. A ventilator is classified as a pressure controller if the ventilator controls the trans-respiratory system _____ (volume, flow, pressure).

30. A positive pressure ventilator applies pressure _____ (inside, outside of) the chest to expand the lungs and it is the type of ventilator most commonly used today.

31. Negative pressure ventilators apply subatmospheric pressure _____ (inside, outside of) the chest to inflate the lungs.

32. For ventilators that are pressure controlled, exhalation occurs when the _____ (positive, negative, positive or negative) pressure ceases.

33. In mechanical ventilation, exhalation is typically due to the _____ (air flow resistance, elastic properties) of the lungs.

34. With a pressure controller, the pressure level that is delivered to the patient _____ (will, will not) vary in spite of changes in the patient's compliance or resistance.

35. With a pressure controller, the volume delivered to the patient _____ (will, will not) vary in conditions of changing compliance or resistance. A _____ (larger, smaller) volume is expected when the compliance is low or the resistance is high.

36. A volume controller allows _____ (flow, pressure, volume) to vary with changes in resistance and compliance, while keeping the _____ (flow, pressure, volume) delivered constant.

37. With a volume controller, the _____ (flow, pressure, volume) becomes _____ (higher, lower) in conditions of decreasing compliance or increasing resistance.

38. Flow controllers allow _____ (time, flow, pressure) to vary with changes in the patient's compliance and resistance while directly measuring and controlling _____ (flow, pressure, volume).

39. With a flow controller, the _____ (flow, pressure, volume) becomes _____ (higher, lower) in conditions of decreasing compliance or increasing resistance.

40. In mechanical ventilation, some ventilators use _____ and _____ to derive the volume delivered.

41. Time controllers are ventilators that measure and control _____ (inspiratory, expiratory, inspiratory and expiratory) time. These ventilators allow _____ (pressure, volume, pressure and volume) to vary with changes in pulmonary compliance and resistance.

42. In conditions of decreasing compliance or increasing resistance, a time controller will cause the _____ (flow, pressure, volume) to _____ (increase, decrease) or the _____ (flow, pressure, volume) to _____ (increase, decrease).

PHASE VARIABLES

43. A ventilator supported breath may be divided into _____ (two, three, four) distinct phases.

44. Describe the phases of a ventilator supported breath.

_____

_____

45. The trigger variable is a factor that determines the _____ (start, end) of _____ (inspiration, expiration).

46. List four factors that can be used as trigger variables during mechanical ventilation.

_____

47. When a ventilator uses change in circuit pressure to initiate inspiration, the mechanical breath is _____ triggered.

48. When a ventilator delivers a breath at a pre-determined time interval, the mechanical breath is _____ triggered.

49. Explain a flow triggered breath.

_____

_____

50. The amount of work needed to initiate or trigger a breath is termed the ventilator _____ (peak airway pressure, peak flow, sensitivity).

51. How should the sensitivity of a ventilator be adjusted to make it easier for the patient to trigger a breath?

_____

_____

52. When one or more variables (pressure, flow, or volume) is not allowed to rise above a preset value during the inspiratory time, it is termed a _____ (trigger, limit, cycle) variable.

53. With a limit variable, inspiration _____ (ends, does not end) when the variable reaches its preset value. The breath delivery _____ (stops, continues) while the variable is held at the fixed, preset value.

54. When the peak pressure reaches a preset value *before* inspiration ends, the breath is _____ (time, pressure, flow, volume) limited.

55. When the volume reaches a preset value *before* inspiration ends, the breath is _____ (flow, pressure, volume, time) limited.

56. With a cycle variable, _____ (inspiration, expiration) ends when a specific cycling variable (i.e., pressure, volume, flow, or time) is reached.

57. When the inspiratory flow ends *because* a preset pressure is reached, the breath is _____ (flow, pressure, volume, time) cycled.

58. When the inspiratory flow ends *because* a preset volume is reached, the breath is _____ (flow, pressure, volume, time) cycled.

59. Baseline variable is a variable that is controlled during the _____ (inspiratory, expiratory) phase or time.

60. Give two examples of baseline variables.

    _____

61. Conditional variables are defined as patterns of variables that are controlled by the _____ (ventilator, patient) during the ventilatory cycle or by the _____ (ventilator, patient) during the spontaneous breathing cycle.

62. Name four conditional variables during mechanical ventilation.

    _____

    _____

OUTPUT WAVEFORMS

63. Name three basic output waveforms during mechanical ventilation.

    _____

    _____

64. The _____ (rectangular, exponential, sinusoidal, oscillating) pressure waveform is characterized by a near instantaneous rise to a peak pressure value that is held constant until the start of exhalation followed by a rapid pressure drop to baseline during exhalation.

65. The _____ (rectangular, exponential, sinusoidal, oscillating) pressure waveform resembles the positive half of a sine wave. These waveforms are produced by ventilators using a _____ (linear, compressor, rotary) driven piston drive mechanism.

66. Name two types of volume waveforms.

_____

67. Name four types of flow waveforms.

_____

_____

ALARM SYSTEMS

68. Input power alarms in mechanical ventilation can be classified as to loss of _____ (electrical, pneumatic power, electrical or pneumatic power).

69. An inappropriate ventilator setting will trigger the _____ (input power, control circuit, output) alarm(s) and this event _____ (allows, does not allow) the clinician to change the input to one that is compatible.

70. What are the five major parameters that output alarms monitor?

_____

71. Airway obstruction is most likely to trigger the _____ (high, low, mean airway, baseline airway) pressure alarm.

72. Circuit disconnection may trigger all of the following pressure alarms *except*:
    A. high pressure alarm.
    B. low pressure alarm.
    C. mean airway pressure alarm.
    D. baseline airway pressure alarm.

73. A _____ (high, low) tidal volume alarm condition may result from over-sedation, circuit disconnection, or apnea.

74. Flow alarms are limited to exhaled _____ (peak flow, tidal volume, minute volume).

75. Time alarms are triggered when the inspiratory time or expiratory time is _____ (too long, too short, too long or too short).

76. Inspired gas alarms alert the clinician to changes in gas _____ (concentration, temperature, concentration or temperature).

77. What are the two common gas analyzers used in mechanical ventilation?

_____

CHAPTER FOUR

OPERATING MODES OF MECHANICAL VENTILATION

NEGATIVE AND POSITIVE PRESSURE VENTILATION

1. Mechanical ventilators deliver flow and volume by creating a _____ pressure gradient between the airway opening and the alveoli.
   A. positive
   B. negative
   C. zero
   D. positive or negative

2. The pressure gradient (difference) between the airway opening and the alveoli is called the:
   A. pleural pressure.
   B. transairway pressure.
   C. transpulmonary pressure.
   D. intrathoracic pressure.

3. Under normal operating conditions, a larger transairway pressure gradient generated by the ventilator creates a _____ (larger, smaller) flow or volume.

4. Negative pressure ventilation creates a transairway pressure gradient by _____ (increasing, decreasing) the alveolar pressures to a level _____ (above, below) the airway opening pressure and the atmospheric pressure.

5. Name two negative pressure ventilators.

   _____

6. An "iron lung" ventilator provides ventilation by creating a negative pressure around the _____ (neck and head, chest cage and abdomen).

7. The tidal volume delivered by a negative pressure ventilator is directly related to the negative pressure gradient.

   (TRUE/FALSE)

8. Disadvantages and complications of the "iron lung" ventilator include _____ and _____.

9. Chest cuirass ventilators are often used in a(n) _____ (acute, home) care facility because they are _____ (easy, difficult) to maintain and _____ (can, cannot) be used to provide ventilation without an artificial airway.

10. When a positive pressure ventilator is used, the tidal volume delivered to the patient is directly related to the positive pressure gradient.

    (TRUE/FALSE)

CYCLING MECHANISM

11. A cycling mechanism is defined as the method a ventilator uses to terminate the _____ (inspiratory, expiratory) phase. Therefore, pressure cycling means the _____ (inspiratory, expiratory) phase is terminated when a preset pressure is reached.

12. When a pressure cycled ventilator is used, the tidal volume delivered varies _____ (directly, inversely) with the lung compliance and _____ (directly, inversely) with the airway resistance.

    In other words, the tidal volume delivered by a pressure cycled ventilator would be decreased in conditions of _____ (high, low) compliance or _____ (high, low) airway resistance.

13. One advantage of _____ (volume, pressure, flow) cycled ventilation is that the inspiratory pressures can be controlled. For instance, the risk of barotrauma can be reduced by keeping the *mean* airway pressure below _____ cm H_2O.

14. Under normal operating conditions, a volume cycled ventilator terminates the _____ (inspiratory, expiratory) phase when a preset _____ (pressure, tidal volume) has been delivered.

15. The primary advantage of a volume cycled ventilator is that the patient is assured of receiving a preset _____ (inspiratory pressure, tidal volume) under normal operating conditions.

16. A flow cycled ventilator mode terminates the inspiratory phase when the inspiratory _____ (volume, pressure, flow) reaches a predetermined minimum level.

17. A time cycled ventilator terminates the inspiratory phase when a preset _____ (flow rate, inspiratory time, expiratory time) has been reached.

18. Once the high pressure limit is reached, the _____ (inspiratory, expiratory) phase is terminated and the ventilator is cycled to the _____ (inspiratory, expiratory) phase.

19. In conditions leading to persistent increases of peak inspiratory pressure, it is acceptable to increase the high pressure limit to silence the related ventilator alarms.

    (TRUE/FALSE)

20. Explain the reason why the high pressure limit should not be set too high.

21. As you are checking the ventilator and patient, you notice that the peak airway pressure has increased from 35 to 48 cm H_2O. This change may be caused by all of the following conditions *except*:

    A. ventilator circuit air leak.

    B. bronchospasm.

    C. mucus plugs.

    D. atelectasis.

TRIGGERING MECHANISM

22. The triggering mechanism is one that signals the ventilator to begin _____ (inspiration, expiration, inspiratory hold) based on an input. Time triggering is an input that comes from the _____ (ventilator, patient). Pressure or flow triggering is an input that comes from the _____ (ventilator, patient).

23. When the respiratory rate of a ventilator is set at 12 breaths per minute, the time triggering interval for each breath is _____ (2, 3, 5, 10) seconds.

24. A pressure triggered breath is initiated when the patient generates a slight _____ (positive, negative) pressure below the baseline pressure at beginning inspiration.

25. The *baseline* pressure from which the patient generates the inspiratory effort is:

    A. –3 cm H_2O.

    B. 0 cm H_2O.

    C. 3 cm H_2O.

    D. variable depending on the level of PEEP.

26. The sensitivity setting on a ventilator determines how much _____ (positive, negative) pressure the patient must generate to initiate a mechanical breath. A sensitivity setting of –3 cm H_2O would require _____ (more, less) patient effort to trigger the ventilator than a setting of –5 cm H_2O.

27. A flow triggered breath is intended to reduce the _____ (inadvertent PEEP, inspiratory effort, peak inspiratory pressure) imposed on the patient during mechanical ventilation.

28. Flow triggering is not activated when the delivered flow [*from the ventilator*] is _____ (greater than, equal to, less than) the return flow [*to the ventilator*].

29. Flow triggering is activated when the return flow [*to the ventilator*] becomes _____ (greater, less) than the delivered flow [*from the ventilator*]. This flow differential signals to the ventilator that part of the _____ (delivered flow, return flow) is used up by the patient during an inspiratory effort.

OPERATING MODES OF MECHANICAL VENTILATION

30. Each of the 13 ventilator modes described in the textbook is used separately and they are not combined during positive pressure ventilation.

    (TRUE/FALSE)

SPONTANEOUS

31. In the spontaneous mode, the work of breathing is provided by the _____ (ventilator, patient).

POSITIVE END-EXPIRATORY PRESSURE (PEEP)

32. Positive end-expiratory pressure (PEEP) increases the end expiratory or baseline airway pressure to a value greater than _____ (−3, 0, 3) cm H_2O. It is used to manage _____ (hypercapnia, hypoxemia, refractory hypoxemia) caused by _____ (hypoventilation, V/Q mismatch, intrapulmonary shunting).

33. When PEEP is used on spontaneously breathing patients, the airway pressure is called _____.

34. List two major indications for PEEP.

    _____

35. Refractory hypoxemia is present when the PaO_2 is less than _____ mm Hg at an F_IO_2 of greater than _____ percent.

36. PEEP provides positive pressure to the lung parenchyma at the _____ (beginning, end) of the _____ (inspiratory, expiratory) phase. It _____ (increases, decreases) the functional residual capacity by alveolar recruitment, _____ (increases, lowers) the alveolar distending pressure, and improves V/Q mismatch and oxygenation.

37. A patient has been using PEEP at levels between 15 to 18 cm H_2O. The physician asks you to monitor the potential adverse effects caused by PEEP. You would monitor all of the following *except*:
    A. decreased venous return.
    B. increased cardiac output and renal perfusion.
    C. barotrauma.
    D. increased intracranial pressure.

38. Venous return to the _____ (left, right) atrium is influenced by the pressure gradient between the central venous pressure and the negative pleural pressure that surrounds the heart. During PEEP, the pleural pressure becomes _____ (more, less) negative and the pressue gradient will decrease resulting in a(n) _____ (increased, decreased) venous return and cardiac output.

39. The effects of PEEP on the venous return is the same regardless of the compliance characteristic of the patient.

    (TRUE/FALSE)

40. The effects of PEEP on the venous return and cardiac output are _____ (more, less) severe in patients with low lung compliance.

41. The incidence of barotrauma is high when the following measurements are obtained: PEEP greater than _____ cm H_2O, mean airway pressure greater than _____ cm H_2O, peak inspiratory pressure greater than _____ cm H_2O.

42. In patients with normal lung compliance, PEEP may _____ (increase, decrease) the intracranial pressure due to impedance of venous return from the head (superior vena cava).

43. Positive pressure ventilation can _____ (improve, reduce) the blood flow to the kidneys. As a result, the urine output is _____ (increased, decreased) as the kidneys try to correct the _____ (hypervolemic, hypovolemic) condition by _____ (retaining, secreting) fluid.

CONTINUOUS POSITIVE AIRWAY PRESSURE (CPAP)

44. Continuous positive airway pressure (CPAP) is _____ applied to the airway of a patient who is breathing spontaneously.

45. The indications for CPAP are essentially the same as for PEEP with the additional requirement that the patient must have adequate spontaneous ventilation documented by the _____ (pH, $PaCO_2$, PaO_2) measurements.

BI-LEVEL POSITIVE AIRWAY PRESSURE (BIPAP)

46. BiPAP may be used to prevent intubation of the end-stage COPD patients and to support patients with chronic ventilatory failure.

    (TRUE/FALSE)

47. In patients who are breathing spontaneously, the initial IPAP and EPAP may be set at _____ (3, 5, 8) cm H_2O and _____ (3, 5, 8) cm H_2O, respectively, and the backup rate may be set at 2 to 5 breaths _____ (above, below) the patient's spontaneous rate.

48. When BiPAP is used in the timed (control) mode, the rate is usually set slightly _____ (higher, lower) than the patient's spontaneous rate.

49. A BiPAP device can be used as a CPAP device by setting the IPAP and EPAP at the same level.

    (TRUE/FALSE)

50. In general, the IPAP is adjusted in 2 cm H_2O increments to regulate the patient's _____ (oxygenation, acid base balance, alveolar ventilation) and the EPAP is adjusted in 2 cm H_2O increments to regulate the patient's _____ (oxygenation, acid base balance, alveolar ventilation).

CONTROLLED MANDATORY VENTILATION

51. With controlled mandatory ventilation, a patient _____ (can, cannot) increase the ventilator respiratory rate or breath spontaneously.

52. The control mode may be used any time without the use of sedatives, respiratory depressants and neuromuscular blockers.

    (TRUE/FALSE)

53. The control mode is indicated in all of the following conditions *except*:
    A. seizure or another activity that hinders mechanical ventilation.
    B. complete rest for the patient for a period of 24 hours.
    C. crushed chest injury with significant paradoxical chest wall movement.
    D. post-anesthesia recovery.

ASSIST CONTROL (AC)

54. With an assist/control (AC) mode, each control breath generates a _____ (spontaneous, mechanical) tidal volume and each assist breath results in a _____ (spontaneous, mechanical) tidal volume.

55. With an assist/control (AC) mode, if the patient has a stable and regular assist rate of 16/min and the ventilator has a control rate of 12/min, the resultant respiratory rate is _____ (12, 16, 28) breaths per minute.

56. The AC mode is typically used for patients who have a(n) _____ (stable, unstable) respiratory drive and _____ (can, cannot) trigger the ventilator into inspiration. Therefore, the ventilator rate is usually set at 2 to 4 breaths per minute _____ (above, below) the patient's assist rate.

57. The AC mode _____ (allows, does not allow) the patient to control the respiratory rate and therefore the minute volume required to normalize the $PaCO_2$.

58. The potential hazard associated with the assist/control mode is alveolar hypoventilation and respiratory acidosis.

    (TRUE/FALSE)

INTERMITTENT MANDATORY VENTILATION (IMV)

59. Intermittent mandatory ventilation (IMV) is a mode in which the ventilator delivers _____ (assist, control) breaths and allows the patient to breath spontaneously at _____ (a preset, any) tidal volume in between the mandatory breaths.

60. In the IMV mode, if the mandatory breaths are delivered at a rate independent of the patient's spontaneous respiratory rate, breath stacking may be a problem.

    (TRUE/FALSE)

SYNCHRONIZED INTERMITTENT MANDATORY VENTILATION (SIMV)

61. Synchronized intermittent mandatory ventilation (SIMV) is a mode in which the ventilator delivers control (mandatory) breaths to the patient at or near the _____ (beginning, end) of a spontaneous breath.

62. The SIMV mandatory breaths may be either time triggered or patient triggered and these mandatory breaths are delivered to the patient at _____ (regular, variable) intervals.

63. When a patient is breathing spontaneously at a SIMV rate of 12/min, a mandatory breath occurs _____ (at precisely, at or about) every _____ (2, 3, 5, 6, 10) seconds.

64. Synchronized intermittent mandatory ventilation (SIMV) is a mode in which the ventilator delivers _____ (assist, control) breaths and allows the patient to breath spontaneously at _____ (a preset, any) tidal volume in between the mandatory breaths.

65. Since SIMV promotes spontaneous breathing and use of respiratory muscles, all of the following are potential advantages of the SIMV mode *except*:
    A. decreased work of breathing.
    B. preventing atrophy of respiratory muscles.
    C. decreased mean airway pressure.
    D. reduced V/Q mismatch.

MANDATORY MINUTE VENTILATION (MMV)

66. Mandatory minute ventilation (MMV), also called minimum minute ventilation, is a feature of some ventilators that provides a predetermined _____ (peak airway pressure, pressure support level, minute ventilation) when the patient's spontaneous breathing effort becomes _____ (excessive, inadequate).

67. MMV is a feature on some ventilators that helps to prevent _____ (hypocapnia, hypercapnia) due to _____ (excessive, inadequate) spontaneous ventilation.

68. A minute volume maintained by rapid spontaneous respiratory rate and low tidal volume (e.g., distressed patient) may avert the MMV function but at the same time will result in a significant amount of dead space ventilation.

    (TRUE/FALSE)

69. A minute volume maintained by rapid spontaneous respiratory rate and low tidal volume may be avoided by properly setting the _____ (high, low) _____ (tidal volume, respiratory rate) alarm.

PRESSURE SUPPORT VENTILATION (PSV)

70. Pressure support ventilation (PSV) is used to increase the work of spontaneous breathing.

    (TRUE/FALSE)

71. Pressure support is commonly used during the weaning process as it helps to _____ (increase, decrease) the patient's spontaneous tidal volume, _____ (increase, decrease) the spontaneous respiratory rate, and _____ (increase, decrease) the work of breathing.

72. The initial pressure support level may be titrated until the spontaneous tidal volume equals to _____ ml/kg or the spontaneous respiratory rate is less than _____ per minute.

PRESSURE CONTROL VENTILATION (PCV)

73. In pressure control ventilation (PCV), the pressure controlled breaths are _____ (patient, time) triggered and therefore the respiratory rate is _____ (variable, preset).

74. Pressure control ventilation can minimize the _____ (tidal volume, peak inspiratory pressure) while still maintaining adequate oxygenation and ventilation.

75. Since the peak inspiratory pressure during PCV is controlled by the preset pressure limit, the tidal volume delivered to the patient will decrease with _____ (high, low) lung compliance and _____ (high, low) airway resistance.

AIRWAY PRESSURE RELEASE VENTILATION (APRV)

76. Airway pressure release ventilation (APRV) is similar to _____ (assist/control, continuous positive airway pressure, intermittent mandatory ventilation) in that the patient is allowed to breath spontaneously without restriction. During spontaneous exhalation, the PEEP is _____ (increased, decreased) to a level _____ (above, below) the baseline pressure.

77. The pressure release mechanism in APRV simulates an effective _____ (inhalation, exhalation) maneuver.

78. In APRV, the pressure release time is usually between _____ and _____ seconds.

79. During the APRV mode, the patient's tidal volume will decrease in conditions of _____ (high, low) lung compliance and _____ (high, low) airway resistance.

80. In some clinical conditions, APRV can provide effective partial ventilatory support with _____ (higher, lower) peak airway pressure than that provided by the PSV and SIMV modes.

INVERSE RATIO VENTILATION (IRV)

81. Inverse ratio ventilation (IRV) improves oxygenation by all of the following mechanisms *except*:
    A. reduction of intrapulmonary shunting.
    B. improvement of V/Q matching.
    C. increase of dead space ventilation.
    D. increase of alveolar recruitment.

82. IRV tends to cause a _____ (higher, lower) mean airway pressure and development of _____ (atelectasis, intrapulmonary shunting, auto-PEEP).

83. The increase in mean airway pressure and development of auto-PEEP during IRV help to reduce shunting and improve oxygenation in ARDS patients.

    (TRUE/FALSE)

84. During IRV, the increase in MAWP leads to a higher incidence of _____ (intrapulmonary shunting, deadspace ventilation, barotrauma).

85. Sedation and neuromuscular blocking agents are often needed to facilitate ventilation in patients receiving IRV.

    (TRUE/FALSE)

86. Since IRV tends to _____ (increase, decrease) mean airway pressure, create auto-PEEP, and increase the incidence of barotrauma, it is sometimes used with pressure control to reduce the airway pressures.

87. When _____ (pressure control, pressure support) is used with IRV, it is called pressure control inverse ratio ventilation (PC-IRV).

CHAPTER FIVE

TEMPORARY AIRWAYS FOR VENTILATION

INTRODUCTION

1. Esophageal obturator airway, esophageal gastric tube airway, laryngeal mask airway, and pharyngealtracheal lumen airway are used as _____ (temporary, permanent) airways.

ESOPHAGEAL OBTURATOR AIRWAY (EOA)

2. An esophageal obturator airway (EOA) is inserted into the _____ (trachea, esophagus) and it is a _____ (reusable, disposable) tube.

3. The EOA has an opening at the _____ (proximal or top, distal or bottom) end, many small holes near the upper end of the tube and a(n) _____ (open, closed) distal end.

4. Near the distal end of an EOA is a _____ (large, small) cuff which is _____ (inflated, deflated) during use.

5. The _____ (inflated, deflated) cuff prevents air from entering the stomach, and subsequent regurgitation and aspiration.

6. A mask is used in conjunction with the EOA tube to:
    A. prevent gas leak around the patient's face during ventilation.
    B. increase oxygen delivery.
    C. provide positive end-expiratory pressure during ventilation.
    D. provide larger tidal volume during ventilation.

7. The small holes at the hypopharyngeal level of an EOA:
    A. prevent regurgitation and aspiration.
    B. provide ventilation to the lungs.
    C. increase the oxygen level.
    D. reduce the dead space volume.

8. Since an EOA is inserted into the _____ (trachea, esophagus), the cuff at the distal end of the tube must be _____ (inflated, deflated) during use.

9. Prior to insertion, the cuff of an EOA is inflated with _____ (5 to 10, 10 to 20, 20 to 30, 30 to 40) cc of air to check for cuff integrity and leaks.

10. Arrange the following four steps in the proper order of preparing an EOA tube for use: _____ (D, A, B, C) *or* (B, A, C, D) *or* (B, D, A, C)
    A. Lubricate tube with a water-soluable lubricant.
    B. Inflate and test cuff.
    C. Insert tube through opening of a mask.
    D. Deflate cuff.

11. Asphyxia and tracheal damage are severe complications if the cuff of an EOA is _____ (inflated, deflated) while the tube is misplaced in the trachea.

12. Which of the following statements is *true* in regard to the use of EOA?
    A. EOA should be used in awake or semiconscious patients.
    B. EOA should not be used in children under 16 years old or under 5 feet tall.
    C. EOA may be used in patients with known esophageal disease.
    D. EOA may be removed before patient has regained consciousness.

13. The EOA _____ (is, is not) designed to use as an artificial airway for positive pressure ventilation.

14. If the EOA is to be replaced with an endotracheal tube, endotracheal intubation should be performed _____ (after removal of EOA, with EOA in place).

ESOPHAGEAL GASTRIC TUBE AIRWAY (EGTA)

15. The major difference between an EOA and an esophageal gastric tube airway (EGTA) is that an EOA has a(n) _____ (open, closed) distal end and an EGTA has a(n) (open, closed) distal end.

16. The advantage of an EGTA is its capability of relieving gastric distention that may occur during bag to mask ventilation.

    (TRUE/FALSE)

17. With an EGTA, ventilation holes along the proximal end of the tube are _____ (absent, present) and ventilation is provided through the _____ (adapter, mask) by a traditional manual resuscitation bag.

18. Since there are two ports on the ETGA mask, the resuscitation bag must be attached to the _____ (gastric, ventilation) port.

19. Distinct features of EOA and EGTA include: EOA and EGTA are both inserted into the _____ (esophagus, trachea); only _____ (EOA, EGTA) has ventilation holes along its tube; only _____ (EOA, EGTA) has a patent distal end; only _____ (EOA, EGTA) has two ports on the mask.

LARYNGEAL MASK AIRWAY (LMA)

20. The laryngeal mask airway (LMA) resembles a _____ (long, short) endotracheal tube with a _____ (large, small) cushioned oblong-shaped mask on the distal end.

21. With proper care and sterilization, the silicone rubber LMA may be reused up to _____ (10, 20, 30, 40, 50) times.

22. A properly inserted LMA provides a seal over the _____ (vocal cords, esophagus, trachea, laryngeal opening) and it _____ (is, is not) necessary for the LMA to enter the larynx or trachea.

23. LMA can withstand positive pressures of up to _____ (10, 20, 30, 40) cm H_2O.

24. LMA is suitable to use during resuscitation in the _____ (conscious, unconscious) patient with _____ (active, absent) glossopharyngeal and laryngeal reflexes.

25. Uses of LMA include: LMA intubation _____ (is, is not) a suitable option following failed endotracheal intubaion attempts; LMA _____ (may, may not) be used in infants and children; LMA provides _____ (higher, lower) work of breathing than an endotracheal tube.

26. LMA _____ (is, is not) capable of protecting an airway from the effects of regurgitation and aspiration.

27. Since LMA can withhold pressures only up to _____ (10, 20, 30) cm H_2O, a leak may occur during high airway pressure situations. Patients with _____ (high, low) airway resistance or _____ (high, low) lung compliance should use an endotracheal tube.

28. The reusable LMA is made with _____ (silicone, polyvinyl chloride).

29. For most adults, size _____ (3, 4, 5, 6) LMA should be used for female and size _____ (3, 4, 5, 6) for male.

30. The standard cuff pressure for an LMA is _____ (20, 30, 40, 50, 60) cm H_2O and it is adjusted accordingly to decrease the intracuff pressure.

31 to 37. Write in the appropriate size of LMA for each respective patient group.

	SIZE	PATIENT GROUP
31.	_____	Neonates and infants up to 5 kg
32.	_____	Infants between 5 and 10 kg
33.	_____	Infants and children between 10 and 20 kg
34.	_____	Children between 20 and 30 kg
35.	_____	Children over 30 kg and small adults
36.	_____	Normal and large adults
37.	_____	Larger adults

38. LMA is inserted _____ (with, without) a laryngoscope through the mouth and advanced along the hard palate. It is then further advanced to the _____ (posterior pharynx, vocal cords) and turned toward the _____ (pharynx, esophagus, trachea and larynx).

39. The LMA may be removed when the patient is _____ (anesthesized, awake, anesthesized or awake).

40. List at least three complications that may occur during removal of LMA.

_____

41. Rotation or turning of the LMA may cause misplacement of the mask and result in gastric insufflation and air leakage from the mask seal.
    (TRUE/FALSE)

42. Reusable LMAs are sterilized by _____ (liquid sterilizing agent, steam autoclave, radiation).

PHARYNGEALTRACHEAL LUMEN AIRWAY (PTLA)

43. Pharyngealtracheal lumen airway (PTLA) is a combination of _____ and _____ in one unit.

44. PTLA is inserted into the _____ (esophagus, trachea, esophagus or trachea).

45. There _____ (is one, are two) cuff(s) on the PTLA.

46. On the PTLA, a proximal latex pharyngeal cuff holds _____ (15, 100) cc of air and a PVC cuff near the distal end of the tube holds _____ (15, 100) cc of air.

47. Lumen A is used to provide ventilation when the PTLA tube enters the _____ (esophagus, trachea) and the _____ (proximal, distal) cuff seals off the _____ (esophagus, trachea).

48. Lumen B is used to provide ventilation when the PTLA tube enters the _____ (esophagus, trachea) and the _____ (proximal, distal) cuff seals off the _____ (esophagus, trachea).

49. PTLA is inserted _____ (with, without, with or without) a laryngoscope.

50. PTLA is properly inserted once the black rings on the tube lie opposite the _____.

51. After insertion of the PTLA, the _____ (distal, proximal, distal and proximal) cuff(s) are inflated immediately.

52. Since PTLA is more likely to enter the _____ (esophagus, trachea) during blind intubation, ventilation through the PTLA should be done via lumen _____ (A, B) first.

53. When the distal end of PTLA is in the _____ (esophagus, trachea), air goes through the side ports, becomes trapped between the cuffs, and it is forced into the trachea.

54. If ventilation via lumen A is poor, lumen B should be used to provide ventilation as the distal end of PTLA may be in the _____ (esophagus, trachea).

55. If ventilation is poor with lumens A and B, a cuff leak may be present and this problem may be corrected by inflating the _____ (distal, proximal) cuff with more air.

56. Complications with PTLA are related to either hemodynamic stress or air leaks.

(TRUE/FALSE)

CHAPTER SIX

AIRWAY MANAGEMENT IN MECHANICAL VENTILATION

INTUBATION

1. Endotracheal (ET) intubation is done by placing an ET tube inside the trachea through the _____ (mouth, nostril, mouth or nostril).

2. _____ (Tracheostomy, Tracheotomy) is a surgical procedure that creates an airway opening by cutting into the trachea whereas _____ (tracheostomy, tracheotomy) is the opening thus created.

3. Compared to an endotracheal tube, a tracheostomy tube is _____ (shorter, longer) and provides closer access to the lower airways.

4. In most emergency situations, _____ (endotracheal intubation, tracheotomy) is the preferred procedure to establish an artificial airway.

5. The decision to perform endotracheal intubation versus tracheotomy is based on the patient's _____ (admitting diagnosis, expected duration of needs, age and weight).

6. Mr. Lang is admitted to the intensive care unit for severe head and chest injuries. He is expected to require mechanical ventilation for the duration and his prognosis is critical. Based on this information, a(n) _____ (endotracheal, tracheostomy) tube is indicated.

7. The indications for endotracheal intubation include all of the following *except* to:
   A. prevent aspiration.
   B. alleviate airway obstruction.
   C. remove secretions.
   D. correct respiratory alkalosis.

8 to 11. Match the indications for artificial airway with the respective examples. Use each answer only once.

INDICATION	EXAMPLES
8. Relief of airway obstruction	A. Loss of swallow or gag reflex
9. Protection of the airway	B. Excessive secretions
10. Facilitation of suctioning	C. Epiglottitis
11. Support of ventilation	D. Mechanical ventilation

COMMON ARTIFICIAL AIRWAYS IN MECHANICAL VENTILATION

12. _____ (Oral intubation, Nasal intubation, Tracheotomy) is easy to perform and it is the artificial airway of choice in emergency situations.

13. The _____ (largest, smallest) endotracheal tube that is appropriate to the patient's size should be used because it offers _____ (more, less) air flow resistance and imposes _____ (more, less) work of breathing on the patient.

14. In comparison to nasal intubation, oral intubation:
    A. is less likely to cause gagging.
    B. produces less secretions.
    C. is better tolerated by the patient.
    D. allows passage of a larger ET tube.

15. Which of the following is *not* associated with nasal intubation?
    A. use of a smaller ET tube
    B. easy to insert
    C. potential of sinusitis
    D. easy to suction secretions

16. A tracheostomy tube allows the patient to eat and drink with the tracheostomy cuff properly _____ (inflated, deflated).

17. Infection is most likely to occur in patients whose artificial airway is provided by a(n) _____ (nasal ET tube, oral ET tube, tracheostomy tube). _____ (Good handwashing, Aseptic, Sterile) technique must be followed to minimize the incidence of infection.

INTUBATION PROCEDURE

18. Which of the following supplies is considered optional for intubating and managing an oral endotracheal tube?
    A. laryngoscope handle and blade
    B. 10 cc syringe
    C. tape
    D. stylet

19. The laryngoscope handle is typically held by the _____ (left, right) hand.

20. A laryngoscope blade comes _____ (straight only, curved only, straight or curved) and it ranges in size from _____ to _____.

21. The Miller blade is a _____ (curved, straight) blade and it is used to lift up the _____ during intubation.

22. The MacIntosh blade is a _____ (curved, straight) blade and its tip is placed in an area called the _____ during intubation.

23. The epiglottis _____ (is, is not) visible through the mouth when a straight blade is used because the straight blade is placed under the epiglottis and _____ (part of the, the entire) soft tissue structure is lifted up anteriorly.

24. The tip of a curved blade rests at the vallecula and it lifts the tongue only. Therefore, the epiglottis _____ (is, is not) visible through the mouth when a curved blade is used properly.

25. During intubation, a _____ (straight, curved) blade lifts the tongue *and* epiglottis upward to expose the vocal cord and related structures, whereas a _____ (straight, curved) blade lifts the tongue only.

26. A _____ (straight, curved) blade works better in patients with short necks, high or rigid larynxes, or obsesity.

27. The tip of a curved blade can be positioned at the vallecula by advancing to the base of the _____.

28. Endotracheal tubes come in sizes ranging from _____ to _____ and each size refers to the _____ (internal, external) diameter of the tube in millimeters (mm).

29. What is the purpose of the radiopaque line implanted along the length of an ET tube?

_____

30. When intubating a spontaneously breathing patient, the ET tube is advanced into the trachea during _____ (inspiratory, expiratory) efforts when the vocal cords are opened wide.

31. A syringe with a capacity of _____ cc or larger is used to test the pilot balloon before intubation and to inflate the cuff after intubation.

32. After successful intubation, the cuff of an ET tube is inflated to _____ (provide ventilation, prevent air leak, apply pressure on the tracheal wall).

33. A(n) _____ (oil-based, water-soluble, petroleum-based) lubricant is used to lubricant the distal end of the ET tube for easy insertion into the trachea.

34. List two adverse outcomes that may occur if the ET tube is not secured properly.

_____

35. A flexible stylet inside an endotracheal tube is required for successful oral intubation and it is often used in nasal intubation.

(TRUE/FALSE)

36. Magill forceps are used to perform _____ (oral intubation, nasal intubation, tracheotomy).

37 to 40. Match the patients with the estimated size of ET tubes. Use *only four* of the answers provided.

PATIENT	ESTIMATED SIZE
37. 800-gm neonate	A. 1 mm I.D.
38. 4000-gm neonate	B. 2.5 mm I.D
39. 8-year-old child	C. 4.0 mm I.D.
40. Adult female	D. 5.0 mm I.D
	E. 6.5 mm I.D.
	F. 8.0 mm I.D.
	G. 9.0 mm I.D.
	H. 10 mm I.D.

41. Given: Estimated ET Tube Size = 4.5 + (Age/4). For a 10-year-old child, the estimated ET tube size would be:
A. 5 mm I.D.
B. 6 mm I.D.
C. 7 mm I.D.
D. 8 mm I.D.

42. During an intubation attempt, the pulse oximetry (SpO_2) reading drops from 95% to 83% and the cardiac monitor shows persistent arrhythmias. This condition is most likely caused by:
A. excessive ET tube size.
B. prolonged intubation attempt.
C. incorrect head position.
D. cardiac arrest.

43. When a patient develops severe hypoxia and arrhythmias during an intubation attempt, all of the following steps should be done *except*:
A. remove blade and ET tube from mouth.
B. provide ventilation.
C. provide oxygenation.
D. provide precordial thump.

44. During oral intubation, the laryngoscope handle and blade should be _____ (pried against the upper teeth, lifted anteriorly to the patient) to clear the tongue and attached soft tissues.

45. Immediately after intubation, bilateral breath sounds are checked _____ (before, after) inflating the ET tube cuff.

46. During nasal intubation, the ET tube is inserted through the nostril and then guided by the _____ (hemostat, fingers, Magill forceps) into the trachea.

47. "Blind" intubation is done by inserting the ET tube into the _____ (mouth, nostril) and advancing it slowly during spontaneous _____ (inspiratory, expiratory) efforts. When air movement is heard through the ET tube, it indicates that the distal end of the ET tube is near the _____ (esophagus, trachea).

48. After intubation, correct placement of the ET tube should be confirmed by checking the bilateral breath sounds and:
    A. distance marking on the ET tube.
    B. chest radiograph.
    C. lateral neck radiograph.
    D. bowel sounds.

49. Esophageal intubation is a(n) _____ (insignificant, grave) error as it can lead to _____ (pneumothorax, cardiac arrest, aspiration). This problem can be avoided by making sure that the ET tube passes through the _____ (area below the tongue, vocal cords, larynx) under direct vision.

50. Indications of successful ET intubation include all of the following *except*:
    A. presence of bilateral breath sounds
    B. presence of CO_2 in expired gas
    C. presence of condensations on ET tube
    D. presence of vocal sounds

51. Bilateral breath sounds should be checked by placing the stethoscope diaphragm along the _____ (anterior aspect of the chest, mid-axillary line).

52. Breath sounds should not be checked at the anterior chest locations close to the trachea since air flow in the esophagus (i.e., in esophageal intubation) can give false "breath sounds" in neonates and thin adults.

    (TRUE/FALSE)

53. In the absence of obvious lung pathology (e.g., atelectasis, consolidation, pleural effusion), uneven bilateral breath sounds may suggest _____ (esophageal, main-stem) intubation.

54. For adult patients, the tip of an ET tube should be about _____ (0.5, 1.5, 3.5) inches _____ (above, below) the carina.

55. Which of the following is *not* an adverse effect of unrecognized esophageal intubation?
    A. hyperventilation
    B. tissue and cerebral hypoxia
    C. vomiting
    D. aspiration

56. If the vocal cords are not seen or cannot be identified during intubation, the ET tube _____ (*may be, must not be*) inserted.

MANAGEMENT OF ENDOTRACHEAL AND TRACHEOSTOMY TUBES

57. _____ (Endotracheal, Tracheostomy) tubes are secured by using adhesive tape or harness and the _____ (endotracheal, tracheostomy) tubes are secured by tying a string to the two openings on the collar.

58. Since the estimated capillary perfusion pressure in the trachea is about _____ (10, 20, 30) cm H_2O, the *maximum* ET tube cuff pressure should not exceed _____ (5, 15, 25) cm H_2O to allow adequate capillary perfusion in the trachea. For patients with _____ (hypertension, hypotension), the cuff pressure should be kept even lower to compensate for the _____ (increased, reduced) capillary flow.

59. Cuff pressure that is _____ (greater, less) than the capillary perfusion pressure in the trachea may cause ischemic injury and tissue necrosis.

60. The _____ (minimal leak technique, minimal occlusion volume) is obtained by slowly _____ (inflating, deflating) the cuff to a point at which no air leak is heard at _____ (end-inspiration, end-expiration) of a mechanical breath.

61. The _____ (end-inspiration, end-expiration) point is used because the trachea reaches its maximal diameter at this point.

62. The _____ (minimal leak technique, minimal occlusion volume) is done by _____ (inflating, deflating) the cuff until the leak stops and then removing a small amount of air until a *slight* leak can be heard at _____ (end-inspiration, end-expiration).

63. Endotracheal suctioning should be done regularly and frequently because it seldomly causes mucosal damage, suction-induced hypoxemia and arrhythmias.

    (TRUE/FALSE)

64. Endotracheal suctioning should be done when rales or crackles are heard, or when secretions are visible in the ET tube.

    (TRUE/FALSE)

65. The level of vacuum pressure should be kept below _____ (50, 100, 150) mm Hg to minimize mucosal damage to the tracheal wall.

66. Describe how to avoid suction-induced hypoxemia.

EXTUBATION

67. In addition to blood gases, muscle strengths, and general cardiopulmonary signs, the rapid breathing index can be a useful indicator of readiness for extubation. It is calculated by: (f = frequency, V_T = spontaneous tidal volume)

    A. $f + V_T$.

    B. $f - V_T$.

    C. $f \times V_T$.

    D. f / V_T.

68. A rapid breathing index of _____ (more, less) than 100/min/L is highly predictive of successful extubation outcome.

69. The f and V_T measurements should be taken as soon as the patient is taken off ventilatory support.

    (TRUE/FALSE)

70. Other criteria that are useful for predicting successful extubation outcome include: spontaneous minute ventilation less than _____ L/min, PaO_2/F_IO_2 more than _____ mm Hg, maximal inspiratory pressure greater than _____ cm H_2O, vital capacity greater than _____ ml/kg, and absence of cardiopulmonary problems.

71. A (P0.1/MIP) ratio of _____ (0.9 or lower, 0.9 or higher) has great predictive value of successful extubation. (P0.1/MIP = occlusion pressure at 0.1 sec to maximal inspiratory pressure)

72. A 68-year-old COPD patient extubated himself and you are asked to evaluate this patient for possible reintubation. Based on the clinical predictors for reintubation listed below, you would recommend that the patient _____ since he has met _____ of the predictors.

UNFAVORABLE CLINICAL PREDICTOR

---

(1) SIMV rate = 10/min

(2) Most recent pH = 7.33

(3) Most recent PaO_2/F_IO_2 = 160 mm Hg

(4) Highest heart rate in the past 24° = 130/min

(5) Patient's diagnosis is COPD, CHF, and renal failure

(6) Patient is alert

(7) Patient is on ventilator due to ventilatory failure

A. be reintubated, 3

B. be reintubated, 5

C. not be reintubated, 3

D. not be reintubated, 5

COMPLICATIONS OF ENDOTRACHEAL INTUBATION

73. Which of the following is *not* a potential complication during intubation?
    A. trauma to teeth and soft tissues
    B. hoarseness
    C. vomiting and aspiration
    D. hypoxia and arrhythmias

74. Which of the following is *not* a potential complication while the patient is intubated?
    A. loss of coughing reflex
    B. aspiration from feeding
    C. main-stem intubation
    D. inadverent extubation

75. Which of the following is *not* a potential complication immediately after extubation?
    A. aspiration
    B. laryngospasm
    C. vomiting
    D. laryngeal and subglottic edema

76. Which of the following is *not* a potential long-term complication some time after extubation?
    A. trauma to teeth and soft tissues
    B. laryngeal stenosis
    C. tracheal inflammation, dilation, and stenosis
    D. vocal cord paralysis

77. Esophageal intubation is often committed by inexperienced practitioners.

    (TRUE/FALSE)

78. Excessive stimulation of the _____ (phrenic, vagus, medial supraclavicular) nerve during intubation attempt can cause bradycardia.

79. While the patient is intubated, kinking of an ET tube leads to _____ (high, low) peak airway pressure and _____ (increased, reduced) air flow.

80. The distance marking on the ET tube (e.g., 22 cm or 26 cm) is used in reference to the patient's _____ (lips, nares, lips or nares).

81. Extubation should be done when the patient is either deeply anesthesized, or preferably, semi-conscious because laryngospasm usually occurs as a result of extubation when the patient is fully awake.

    (TRUE/FALSE)

82. Stridor is the _____ (harsh or high-pitched sound, gentle or low-pitched sound) heard during spontaneous breathing. It is heard when the upper airway is _____ (partially, completely) obstructed.

83. The best way to avoid long-term complications (e.g., laryngeal stenosis, tracheal inflammation) following use of artificial airway is to:
    A. use the largest ET tube possible.
    B. practice proper intubation technique.
    C. suction airway frequently.
    D. provide proper airway care.

CHAPTER SEVEN

NONINVASIVE POSITIVE PRESSURE VENTILATION

TERMINOLOGY

1. Noninvasive positive pressure ventilation refers to a mechanical ventilation strategy without the use of _____ .

2. Continuous positive airway pressure (CPAP) _____ (does, does not) include mechanical breaths and the work of breathing is entirely assumed by the _____ (ventilator, patient).

3. Bilevel positive airway pressure (Bilevel PAP) can be used to provide _____ (one, two, one or two) levels of airway pressure.

4. When bilevel PAP is used, the peak airway pressure is controlled by the _____ (IPAP, EPAP) setting and the CPAP or PEEP level is controlled by the _____ (IPAP, EPAP) setting.

PHYSIOLOGICAL EFFECTS OF NPPV

5. If a larger tidal volume is desired, the _____ (IPAP, EPAP) level should be _____ (increased, decreased).

6. The functional residual capacity can be increased by increasing the _____ (IPAP, EPAP) level.

7. _____ (IPAP, EPAP) relieves upper airway obstruction with its splinting action.

8. List two or more laboratory parameters that may be used as titration endpoints for the IPAP and EPAP levels.

USE OF CONTINUOUS POSITIVE AIRWAY PRESSURE (CPAP)

9. CPAP provides positive airway pressure during the _____ (inspiratory phase, expiratory phase, entire spontaneous breath) and it _____ (does, does not) include any mechanical breaths.

10. Compared to mechanical ventilation, CPAP imposes _____ (more, less) work of breathing on the patient.

11. CPAP is considered a noninvasive ventilation strategy because it _____ (does, does not) require an artificial airway, uses a nasal or facial mask, and requires airway pressures.

12. When the inspiratory pressure and expiratory pressure of a bilevel positive airway pressure device are set at the same level, _____ (IPPB, CPAP, PEEP) results.

13. CPAP is the treatment of choice for _____ (central, obstructive, mixed) sleep apnea without significant carbon dioxide retention.

14. CPAP should not be used to manage apnea due to _____ (airflow obstruction, neuromuscular causes).

15. Sleep apnea is defined as a temporary pause in breathing that lasts at least _____ (5, 10, 20) seconds during sleep.

16. The cause of obstructive sleep apnea is severe _____ (lung volume restriction, airflow obstruction) during sleep.

17. Prosthetic mandibular advancement, tonsillectomy, uvulopalatopharyngoplasty, weight reduction gastric surgery, and CPAP are some strategies for the management of _____ (central sleep apnea, obstructive sleep apnea, mixed apnea).

USE OF BILEVEL POSITIVE AIRWAY PRESSURE (BILEVEL PAP)

18. Bilevel PAP has an inspiratory positive airway pressure (IPAP) setting that provides _____ and an expiratory positive airway pressure (EPAP) level that functions as _____ .

19. List two major indications for bilevel PAP when it is used as an adjunct to provide mechanical ventilation.

_____

20. For patients with hypoxemic respiratory failure, refractory hypoxemia is present when the PaO_2/F_IO_2 ratio is _____ (more than, less than) 200.

21. Which of the following is *not* an indication for NPPV?
    A. reduction of respiratory workload in obesity
    B. acute respiratory failure
    C. chronic ventilatory failure
    D. acute hypercapnic exacerbations of COPD

22. Contraindications for NPPV include all of the following *except*:
    A. apnea
    B. inability to handle secretions
    C. facial trauma
    D. claustrophobia
    E. acute respiratory acidosis

23. Patients who are unable to handle secretions should not be placed on NPPV because _____ (hypoventilation, aspiration, respiratory failure, apnea) can be a potential problem without an artificial airway.

COMMON INTERFACES FOR CPAP AND BILEVEL PAP

24. In NPPV, the external device that connects the ventilator tubing to the patient's nose, mouth, or face is called a(n) _____.

25. List three common interfaces used in NPPV.

    _____

26. When a nasal mask is used during NPPV, it _____ (must have a tight seal, may have a minor leak, may have a large leak).

27. In selecting a new nasal mask, a common error is selecting one that is too _____ (large, small) for the patient.

28. If air leak around the nasal mask is significant after trying on different sizes, the _____ (nasal pillows, facial mask, endotracheal tube, laryngeal mask airway) should be considered.

29. Another problem with nasal mask is air leak through the _____ , particularly when the positive pressure level is high.

30. Immediately after setting up the nasal mask, _____ (pulse oximetry, blood gas) is done to check for improvement in oxygenation. This should be followed by _____ (pulse oximetry, blood gas) for fine tuning the pressure settings.

31. List two advantages of using nasal mask in NPPV.

    _____

32. List two disadvantages of using a nasal mask in NPPV.

    _____

33. Facial mask is an interface used in NPPV that covers the patient's nose and mouth area.

    (TRUE/FALSE)

34. Since a facial mask covers the patient's nose and mouth, list two potentially harmful problems in using this interface.

    _____

35. Besides regurgitation and aspiration, and asphyxiation, list three disadvantages of using a facial mask in NPPV.

_____

36. Nasal pillows resemble a small nasal mask and it consists of two small cushions that fit under the _____ . It is commonly used during _____ (bilevel PAP, CPAP, IPPB) therapy.

37. Since nasal pillows can withstand airway pressures of up to _____ (10, 20, 30, 40) cm H_2O, they are _____ (more, less) effective than the nasal and facial masks.

POTENTIAL PROBLEMS WITH INTERFACES

38. Which of the following is not a strategy to reduce air leaks through an interface during NPPV?
    A. adjusting headgear
    B. using chin strap
    C. reducing pressure setting
    D. using spacers or foam pads
    E. trying another size or mask

39. Which of the following is not effective in minimizing skin breakdown or irritation during NPPV?
    A. adjusting or trying another headgear
    B. using chin strap
    C. using spacers, foam pads or topical ointments
    D. trying a different cleaning solution
    E. resizing mask or trying another mask

TITRATION OF CONTINUOUS POSITIVE AIRWAY PRESSURE

40. The _initial_ CPAP setting is typically _____ (2, 4, 6, 8) cm H_2O.

41. If the bilevel PAP device does not have a separate CPAP control, a CPAP level of 4 cm H_2O may be obtained by setting the:
    A. IPAP at 4 cm H_2O and EPAP at 0 cm H_2O.
    B. IPAP at 8 cm H_2O and EPAP at 4 cm H_2O.
    C. IPAP and EPAP at 4 cm H_2O.
    D. IPAP at 0 cm H_2O and EPAP at 4 cm H_2O.

42. The CPAP level is fine tuned by observing the following parameters:
    A. SpO_2 readings and number of apnea episodes.
    B. number of apnea episodes.
    C. PCO_2 and SpO_2 readings.
    D. PO_2 and SpO_2 readings.

TITRATION OF BILEVEL POSITIVE AIRWAY PRESSURES

43. The *initial* bilevel PAP settings are typically IPAP at _____ (0, 4, 8, 12, 16) cm H_2O and EPAP at _____ (0, 4, 8, 12, 16) cm H_2O.

44. The IPAP maximum time should be set _____ second longer than the patient's actual inspiratory time and the IPAP maximum time should not be longer than _____ % of the respiratory cycle.

45. The IPAP level is increased in _____ cm H_2O increments to provide more _____.

46. The EPAP level is increased in _____ cm H_2O increments to _____.

47. If poor synchronization occurs during NPPV, check for _____ (air leaks, oxygen flow, pressure settings) or alter _____ (EPAP level, IPAP level, IPAP maximum time).

48. Oxygen should be added if the baseline oxygen saturation remains low with appropriate IPAP and EPAP settings.

    (TRUE/FALSE)

49. IPAP or EPAP level should not be set beyond patient tolerance.

    (TRUE/FALSE)

CHAPTER EIGHT

INITIATION OF MECHANICAL VENTILATION

INDICATIONS

1. Mechanical ventilation is indicated in all of the following conditions *except*:
   A. acute or impending ventilatory failure.
   B. severe hypoxemia.
   C. prophylatic ventilatory support.
   D. metabolic acid base imbalance.

2. Acute ventilatory failure is defined as a _____ (gradual, sudden) increase of the _____ ($PaCO_2$, PaO_2) to greater than 50 mm Hg with an accompanying respiratory _____ (acidosis, alkalosis).

3. In patients with chronic CO_2 retention, mechanical ventilation may be indicated when the $PaCO_2$ is more than 10 mm Hg _____ (above, below) the patient's baseline value with an accompanying respiratory _____ (acidosis, alkalosis), generally _____ (more, less) than 7.30.

4. Impending ventilatory failure becomes evident when the _____ (pH, $PaCO_2$, PaO_2) shows a _____ (acute, gradual) and persistent increase.

5. At the early stage of impending ventilatory failure, the $PaCO_2$ value may be normal or low due to _____ (renal, respiratory) compensation for the gas exchange deficiencies. This compensation is characterized by alveolar _____ (hyperventilation, hypoventilation).

6. Five clinical signs have been used to indicate the development of impending ventilatory failure. Complete the table below to define the threshold for each clinical sign.

CLINICAL SIGN	IMPENDING VENTILATORY FAILURE LIKELY WHEN
Spontaneous V_T	Less than _____ ml/kg
Spontaneous rate	_____ (Greater than, Less than) 25 to 35/min
Spontaneous minute volume	Greater than _____ liters
Vital capacity	Less than _____ ml/kg
Maximal inspiratory pressure	Less than _____ cm H_2O

7. Severe hypoxemia is present when the PaO_2 is less than _____ on _____ or more of oxygen or less than 40 mm Hg at any F_IO_2.

8. When the $P(A-a)O_2$ measurement is used to evaluate a patient's oxygenation status, every 50 mm Hg difference in $P(A-a)O_2$ approximates _____ (2, 5, 10) percent of intrapulmonary shunt. (At an F_IO_2 of 100%)

9. Given: $PAO_2 = 260$ mm Hg, $PaO_2 = 70$ mm Hg.   What is the calculated $P(A-a)O_2$ and the estimated shunt percent?
   A. $P(A-a)O_2 = 150$ mm Hg, 3% shunt
   B. $P(A-a)O_2 = 150$ mm Hg, 6% shunt
   C. $P(A-a)O_2 = 190$ mm Hg, 6% shunt
   D. $P(A-a)O_2 = 190$ mm Hg, 8% shunt

10. The PAO_2 can be calculated by using the simplified alveolar air equation as shown below.
    A. $PAO_2 = (P_B - PH_2O) \times F_IO_2$
    B. $PAO_2 = (P_B - PH_2O) \times F_IO_2 - PaCO_2$
    C. $PAO_2 = (P_B - PH_2O) \times F_IO_2 - (PaCO_2/R)$
    D. $PAO_2 = (P_B - PH_2O) \times F_IO_2 - (PaCO_2 \times 1.5)$

11. Prophylatic ventilatory support is provided in clinical conditions in which the risk of pulmonary complications, ventilatory failure, or oxygenation failure is relatively low.

    (TRUE/ FALSE)

CONTRAINDICATIONS

12. Positive pressure ventilation is contraindicated in:
    A. pleural effusion.
    B. hemothorax.
    C. tension pneumothorax.
    D. all of the above.

13. Positive pressure ventilation may be used to ventilate patients with tension pneumothorax after placement of a _____ to relieve the pleural _____ (fluid, blood, pressure).

14. Initiation of mechanical ventilation is sometimes withheld:
    A. on patient's request.
    B. in cases of medical futility.
    C. to reduce or terminate a patient's pain and suffering.
    D. all of the above.

15. Medical futility means that medical intervention is most likely _____ (useful, useless) based on previous experience in similar cases.

INITIAL VENTILATOR SETTINGS

16. _____ (Full, Partial) ventilatory support (i.e., control mode, assist/control mode, high SIMV rate) is necessary if the patient is not breathing spontaneously between mechanical breaths.

17. Partial ventilatory support is indicated if the patient is _____ (able, unable) to assume _____ (part, all) of the work of breathing.

18. The initial respiratory rate (frequency) should be the estimated number of breaths per minute needed to provide _____ (hyperventilation, eucapneic ventilation, hyperoxia).

19. Eucapneic ventilation is achieved when the patient's $PaCO_2$ is at _____ (40 mm Hg, the patient's normal value).

20. The initial respiratory rate on a ventilator may be set between _____ and _____ breaths per minute.

21. High respiratory rates (e.g., 20 or more breaths/min) during positive pressure ventilation may not allow adequate time for _____ (inspiration, expiration). This in turn may lead to development of _____ (hyperventilation, hypoventilation, auto-PEEP).

22. List three conditions that may lead to development of auto-PEEP.

    _____

23. The respiratory rate (frequency) setting on a ventilator is the primary control used to alter a patient's _____ (pH, heart rate, PaO_2, $PaCO_2$).

24. In general, the respiratory rate setting on a ventilator should be _____ (increased, decreased) if the $PaCO_2$ is too high; _____ (increased, decreased) if the $PaCO_2$ is too low.

25. The initial tidal volume setting on the ventilator should be set between _____ and _____ ml/kg of ideal body weight.

26. Occasionally tidal volumes as low as 6 ml/kg are used to provide intentional _____ (hyperventilation, hypoventilation). This type of ventilation (i.e., permissive hypercapnia) is done to minimize the airway pressures and the risk of _____ (hyperventilation, auto-PEEP, barotrauma).

27. Decreasing the tidal volume by 100 to 200 ml is one strategy used to _____ (increase, reduce) the expiratory time requirement and prevent _____ (atelectasis, hypoventilation, air trapping) in COPD patients.

28 to 30. Certain clinical conditions may benefit from lower mechanical tidal volumes (i.e., lower airway pressures). Match the conditions below with the respective examples. Use each answer only once.

CONDITION	EXAMPLES
28. Increase of airway pressure requirement	A. Pneumonectomy
29. Increase of lung compliance	B. ARDS
30. Decrease of lung volumes	C. Emphysema

31. The tidal volume delivered to the patient by the ventilator is usually _____ (higher, lower) than the preset tidal volume due to gas leakage and circuit compressible volume loss.

32. Given: Expired volume = 120 ml; Peak inspiratory pressure at 0 PEEP (Y occlusion) = 30 cm H_2O. Calculate the circuit compression factor.
    A. 2.5 ml/cm H_2O
    B. 3.6 ml/cm H_2O
    C. 4 ml/cm H_2O
    D. 36 ml/cm H_2O

33. Given: Circuit compression factor = 3 ml/cm H_2O; Peak inspiratory pressure (mechanical ventilation) = 50 cm H_2O; PEEP = 10 cm H_2O. Calculate the circuit compression volume at this peak inspiratory pressure and PEEP.
    A. 17 ml
    B. 60 ml
    C. 120 ml
    D. 150 ml

34. Given: Expired tidal volume = 820 ml; Circuit compression volume = 150 ml. What is the corrected tidal volume?
    A. 670 ml
    B. 820 ml
    C. 970 ml
    D. 1070 ml

35. For patients with severe hypoxemia, the initial F_IO_2 may be set at 100%. It should be adjusted until the _____ (PaO_2, $PaCO_2$) is maintained between _____ (80 and 100 mm Hg, 35 to 45 mm Hg) for normal patients but _____ (higher, lower) for patients with chronic CO_2 retention.

36. After the patient has been stabilized, the F_IO_2 should be kept below _____ to avoid oxygen-induced lung injuries.

37. For patients with mild hypoxemia or normal cardiopulmonary functions (e.g., drug overdose, uncomplicated post-operative recovery), the initial F_IO_2 may be set at _____ or at the patient's F_IO_2 prior to mechanical ventilation.

38. For patients with refractory hypoxemia, the initial PEEP level may be set at _____ cm H_2O. Subsequent changes of PEEP should be based on the patient's blood gas results, F_IO_2 requirement, tolerance of PEEP, and cardiovascular responses.

39. The initial I:E ratio is usually kept in a range between _____ to _____. A larger I:E ratio (longer E ratio) may be used on patients needing additional time for exhalation because of the possibility of _____ (atelectasis, air trapping) and auto-PEEP.

40. Occurrence of air trapping during mechanical ventilation may be checked by occluding the _____ (inspiratory, expiratory) port of the ventilator circuit at the _____ (beginning, end) of exhalation. Auto-PEEP is present when the _____ (beginning-expiratory, end-expiratory pressure) does not return to baseline pressure.

41. Inverse I:E ratio has been used to correct refractory hypoxemia in ARDS patients with very _____ (high, low) compliance.

42. In addition to the inspiratory flow rate (peak flow), all of the following ventilator controls may affect the I:E ratio *except*:

    A. respiratory rate.

    B. inspiratory time or inspiratory time %.

    C. minute volume.

    D. PEEP.

43. By increasing the inspiratory flow rate (peak flow), the inspiratory time (I time) becomes _____ (longer, shorter) and the expiratory time (E time) becomes _____ (longer, shorter). [Assume the V_T and RR are kept unchanged]

44. Describe the effects of a decreased inspiratory flow rate on the I time and E time. [Assume the V_T and RR are kept unchanged]

    _____

45. By increasing the tidal volume, the I time becomes _____ (longer, shorter) and the E time becomes _____ (longer, shorter). [Assume the flow rate and RR are kept unchanged]

46. Describe the effects of a smaller tidal volume on the I time and E time. [Assume the flow rate and RR are kept unchanged]

    _____

47. When the flow rate and V_T are kept constant, changes in the RR have little effect on the _____ (I time, E time) but the _____ (I time, E time) varies inversely with the RR change.

48. A higher RR _____ (lengthens, shortens) the E time and a slower RR _____ (lengthens, shortens) the E time. [Assume the flow rate and V_T are kept unchanged]

49. Given: Minute Volume = 12 l/min. Calculate the minimum flow rate needed for an I:E ratio of 1:4.

    A. 30 l/min

    B. 40 l/min

    C. 50 l/min

    D. 60 l/min

50. Given: RR = 12/min. Calculate the I time and the E time for an I:E ratio of 1:3.

    A. I time = 0.75 sec; E time = 4.25 sec

    B. I time = 1 sec; E time = 4 sec

    C. I time = 1.25 sec; E time = 3.75 sec

    D. I time = 1.5 sec; E time = 3.5 sec

51. Given: Desired I:E Ratio = 1:3 Calculate the I time % needed for an I:E ratio of 1:3.

    A. 25%

    B. 33%

    C. 50%

    D. 67%

52. List the four common flow patterns available on adult ventilators.

_____

53. Selection of a flow pattern on the ventilator should be based on the patient's condition and the measureable improvement of the patient's ventilatory and oxygenation status on a selected flow pattern.

(TRUE/FALSE)

VENTILATOR ALARM SETTINGS

54. The low exhaled volume alarm (low volume alarm) is typically used to detect _____ (excessive system pressure, system leak) or _____ (circuit obstruction, circuit disconnection).

55. The low exhaled volume alarm should be set at about _____ (100 ml, 200 ml, 300 ml) _____ (higher, lower) than the _____ (preset, expired) mechanical tidal volume.

56. The low inspiratory pressure alarm is used to detect system leak or circuit disconnection.

(TRUE/FALSE)

57. The low inspiratory pressure alarm should be set at _____ (0 to 10 cm H_2O, 10 to 15 cm H_2O, 15 to 20 cm H_2O) _____ (above, below) the observed peak inspiratory pressure.

58. The high inspiratory pressure alarm (high pressure limit alarm) should be set at _____ (0 to 10 cm H_2O, 10 to 15 cm H_2O, 15 to 20 cm H_2O) _____ (above, below) the observed peak inspiratory pressure.

59. The high inspiratory pressure alarm may be triggered by all of the following conditions _except_:
    A. secretions in the airway.
    B. kinking or bitting of the endotracheal tube.
    C. bronchospasm.
    D. circuit disconnection.

60. Once the high inspiratory pressure is triggered, _____ (inspiration, expiration) is immediately terminated and the ventilator changes to the _____ (inspiratory, expiratory) cycle. As a result, the volume delivered by the ventilator will become _____ (larger, smaller).

61. The apnea alarm should be set with a _____ (5 to 10 seconds, 15 to 20 seconds, 20 to 30 seconds) time delay, with a longer time delay at _____ (higher, lower) ventilator rate.

62. The high respiratory rate alarm (high rate alarm) should be set at _____ (5 to 10 breaths/min, 10 to 15 breaths/min, 15 to 20 breaths/min) _____ (over, below) the observed respiratory rate.

63. Triggering of the high rate alarm shows tachynea and it is a sign of _____ (alveolar hyperventilation, alveolar hypoventilation, respiratory distress).

64. The high F_1O_2 alarm should be set at 5 to 10% _____ (over, below) the analyzed F_1O_2 and the low F_1O_2 alarm should be set at 5 to 10% (over, below) the analyzed F_1O_2.

65 to 71. Match the ventilator parameters with the initial alarm settings. Choose *one* answer from each set of answers provided.

OBSERVED PARAMETER	INITIAL ALARM SETTING
65. Expired volume = 700 ml	A. Low volume alarm = 500 ml
	B. Low volume alarm = 600 ml
	C. Low volume alarm = 800 ml
	D. Low volume alarm = 900 ml
66. Peak airway pressure = 60 cm H_2O	A. Low pressure alarm = 45 cm H_2O
	B. Low pressure alarm = 55 cm H_2O
	C. Low pressure alarm = 65 cm H_2O
	D. Low pressure alarm = 75 cm H_2O
67. Peak airway pressure = 60 cm H_2O	A. High pressure alarm = 45 cm H_2O
	B. High pressure alarm = 55 cm H_2O
	C. High pressure alarm = 65 cm H_2O
	D. High pressure alarm = 75 cm H_2O
68. Ventilator SIMV rate = 8/min	A. Apnea time delay = 5 sec
	B. Apnea time delay = 10 sec
	C. Apnea time delay = 20 sec
	D. Apnea time delay = 30 sec
69. Ventilator SIMV rate = 8/min	A. High rate alarm = 10/min
	B. High rate alarm = 20/min
	C. High rate alarm = 30/min
	D. High rate alarm = 40/min
70. Analyzed F_1O_2 = 50%	A. High F_1O_2 alarm = 35%
	B. High F_1O_2 alarm = 45%
	C. High F_1O_2 alarm = 55%
	D. High F_1O_2 alarm = 65%
71. Analyzed F_1O_2 = 50%	A. Low F_1O_2 alarm = 35%
	B. Low F_1O_2 alarm = 45%
	C. Low F_1O_2 alarm = 55%
	D. Low F_1O_2 alarm = 65%

HAZARDS AND COMPLICATIONS

72 to 75. Match the conditions leading to complications in mechanical ventilation with the respective examples. Use each answer only once.

CONDITION	EXAMPLES
72. Related to positive pressure ventilation	A. Nosocomial pneumonia
73. Related to patient condition	B. Physical and psychologic trauma
74. Related to equipment and supplies	C. Barotrauma
75. Related to medical professionals	D. Circuit disconnection

76. Barotrauma is lung tissue injury or rupture that is caused by alveolar _____ (atelectasis, overdistention).

77. Risk of barotrauma is increased when the airway pressures are high. Complete the table below to define the threshold for each airway pressure.

AIRWAY PRESSURE	INCREASED RISK OF BAROTRAUMA WHEN
Peak airway pressure	Greater than _____ cm H_2O
Plateau pressure	Greater than _____ cm H_2O
Mean airway pressure	Greater than _____ cm H_2O
PEEP	Greater than _____ cm H_2O

78. During mechanical ventilation, development of barotrauma is _____ (more, less) likely in COPD patients due to _____ (fibrosis, air trapping) and _____ (tightened, weakened) lung tissues.

79. Other lung injuries that may occur as a result of positive pressure ventilation include all of the following *except*:

A. pulmonary interstitial emphysema.

B. pulmonary fibrosis.

C. pneumomediastinum.

D. subcutaneous emphysema.

80. Since positive pressure ventilation _____ (increases, decreases) the central venous pressure, the pressure gradient between the right atrium and the venous drainage will be _____ (increased, decreased).

81. A reduced pressure gradient between the right atrium and the venous drainage means a _____ (higher, lower) venous return to the right atrium and _____ (higher, lower) cardiac output.

82. In patients with a competent cardiovascular system, a small drop in venous return may be compensated by _____ (increasing, decreasing) the heart rate and _____ (constricting, dilating) the arterial blood vessels.

83. High airway pressures are more detrimental to the cardiac output in patients with _____ (high, low) lung compliance than those with _____ (high, low) compliance.

CHAPTER NINE

MONITORING IN MECHANICAL VENTILATION

VITAL SIGNS

1. The normal adult heart rate is between _____ and _____ per minute.

2. Tachycardia means a heart rate greater than _____.

3. Tachycardia may be caused by all of the following clinical conditions *except*:
   A. hypoxemia.
   B. hypovolemia.
   C. fever.
   D. hypothermia.

4. Bradycardia means a heart rate less than _____.

5. Bradycardia may be caused by all of the following clinical conditions *except*:
   A. pain and stress.
   B. sinoatrial node malfunction.
   C. obstruction of coronary blood flow.
   D. prolonged suctioning.

6. A patient's blood pressure may be monitored via an indwelling arterial catheter inserted in any of the following arteries *except*:
   A. brachial artery.
   B. popliteal artery.
   C. carotid artery.
   D. radial artery.

7. Fluid overload, vasoconstriction, stress, anxiety, and pain may initially lead to _____ (hypertension, hypotension, cardiac arrest).

8. When hypotension occurs during positive pressure ventilation, it is often associated with _____ (excessive, inadequate) intrathoracic pressure, peak airway pressure, and lung volume.

9. Absolute hypovolemia can lead to _____ (hypertension, hypotension). An example of *absolute* hypovolemia is _____ (severe hemorrhage, shock).

10. Relative hypovolemia can also lead to _____ (hypertension, hypotension). An example of *relative* hypovolemia is _____ (dehydration, sepsis).

11. In general, absolute hypovolemia is related to _____ (excessive, inadequate) circulating volume and it can be corrected by blood or fluid replacement.

12. Relative hypovolemia is related to _____ (excessive, loss of) venous tone. When the venous vessels dilate, the relative amount of circulating volume becomes _____ (excessive, inadequate). Relative hypovolemia can be corrected by treating the cause of venous dilation and *partial* fluid replacement.

13. Hypervolemia and positive pressure ventilation are two causes of hypotension.

    (TRUE/FALSE)

14. The normal spontaneous respiratory rate for adults is _____ breaths per minute.

15. Tachypnea means a(n) _____ (increased, decreased) respiratory rate and it may be an early warning sign of _____ (repiratory alkalosis, respiratory distress).

16. One strategy of weaning from mechanical ventilation is to allow the patient to breathe spontaneously without ventilator assistance. When tachypnea and low tidal volume are observed in a spontaneously breathing patient, it is indicative of _____ (successful, unsuccessful) weaning outcome.

17. _____ (Hyperthermia, Hypothermia) may be caused by conditions which increase a patient's metabolic rate and oxygen utilization. Furthermore, it shifts the oxyhemoglobin dissociation curve to the _____ (right, left) causing a _____ (higher, lower) oxygen saturation at any PaO_2.

18. Hypothermia is *least* likely caused by:
    A. infection.
    B. central nervous system (CNS) problem.
    C. metabolic disorder.
    D. cold exposure.

19. _____ (Hyperthermia, Hypothermia) is sometimes induced in head trauma patients to decrease the patient's basal _____ (respiratory, metabolic) rate.

20. When _____ (hyperthermia, hypothermia) is induced in patients undergoing coronary artery bypass (CAB) surgery, the measured PaO_2 and $PaCO_2$ values are _____ (higher, lower) than the actual values when the sample is collected under _____ (hyperthermic, hypothermic) condition and analyzed at body temperature.

21. For blood gas samples obtained during CAB surgery, temperature corrections to _____ (room temperature, 37°C, patient's core temperature) must be done during blood gas analysis to accurately measure a patient's ventilatory and oxygenation status.

22. Excessive cooling of the _____ (ulnar, phrenic, median) nerves during CAB surgey may lead to _____ (venous admixture, hypoventilation, blood clot) due to _____ (shunting, paralysis of hemidiaphragms, vasoconstriction).

CHEST INSPECTION AND AUSCULTATION

23. Asymmetrical movement of the chest can occur in all of the following conditions *except*:
    A. main-stem intubation.
    B. atelectasis.
    C. consolidation.
    D. tension pneumothorax.

24 to 27. Match the abnormal breath sounds with the related clinical conditions. Use each answer only once.

BREATH SOUND	CONDITIONS
24. Diminished or absent	A. Pulmonary edema
25. Wheezes	B. Atelectasis
26. Inspiratory crackles	C. Excessive secretions
27. Coarse crackles	D. Airway narrowing

28 to 32. Match the lung segments with the surface projections (landmarks) of these segments. Use *only five* of the answers provided.

LUNG SEGMENT	SURFACE PROJECTION
28. Right upper lobe anterior segment	A. Left mid-axillary line about 6 inches below armpit
29. Right middle lobe medial segment	B. Left posterior 6 inches below scapula next to spine
30. Left upper lobe lingula inferior segment	C. Right nipple area (male)
31. Left lower lobe anterior segment	D. Right side under armpit
32. Left lower lobe superior segment	E. Left nipple area (male)
	F. Right anterior chest between clavicle and nipple (male)
	G. Left posterior below scapula next to spine

33. Proper identification of the lung segments based on surface projections is useful in all of the following procedures *except*:
    A. charting and reporting.
    B. intubation and extubation.
    C. chest physiotherapy.
    D. chest auscultation.

34. A cuff leak of the endotracheal tube may be detected by placing the stethoscope diaphragm over the _____ (mouth, trachea, lungs). A moderate leak is present if air movement can be heard _____ (at the beginning, toward the end) of a mechanical breath. If the leak is significant, air movement out of the mouth will become evident.

FLUID BALANCE AND ANION GAP

35. During positive pressure ventilation, the urine output may be decreased due to:
    A. hyperperfusion of the kidneys.
    B. reduction of antidiuretic hormone.
    C. increase of atrial natriuretic hormone.
    D. reduction of cardiac output.

36. Monitoring the urine output is important in the management of fluid balance. Oliguria means _____ (excessive, scanty) urine output and it may indicate _____ (fluid overload, fluid inadequacy).

37. Oliguria may occur as a result of:
    A. kidney malfunction.
    B. increased renal perfusion.
    C. increased fluid intake.
    D. increased cardiac output.

38. Normal urine output is _____ ml/hr.

39. Mr. Jones has a urine output of 200 ml in a 24-hour period. This condition is indicative of fluid overload.

    (TRUE/FALSE)

40. Oliguria is present when the urine output is less than _____ ml/hr, _____ ml in a 24-hour period, or _____ ml in an 8-hour period.

41. Reduction in cardiac output can be directly attributed to _____ (increased, decreased) venous return secondary to positive pressure ventilation and _____ (increased, decreased) intrathoracic pressure.

42. Positive pressure ventilation also causes a(n) _____ (increase, decrease) in the production of antidiuretic hormone (ADH), which _____ (increases, reduces) the urine output.

43. Write in the normal values of the four major electrolytes.

CATION		CONCENTRATION	ANION		CONCENTRATION
Na^+	_____	mEq/L	Cl^-	_____	mEq/L
K^+	_____	mEq/L	HCO_3^-	_____	mEq/L

44. A patient's recent laboratory report reveals the following electrolyte measurements: Na^+ = 133 mEq/L; Cl^- 101 mEq/L; K^+ 3 mEq/L; $HCO3^-$ 23 mEq/L. What is the anion gap? Is it within the normal range?
    A. 12 mEq/L, lower than normal
    B. 15 mEq/L, lower than normal
    C. 12 mEq/L, higher than normal
    D. 15 mEq/L, higher than normal

45. Mr. Lawson has the following blood gas and electrolyte results: pH = 7.20, $PaCO_2$ = 35 mm Hg, HCO_3^- = 13 mEq/L, Na^+ = 140 mEq/L; Cl^- 114 mEq/L. Based on his anion gap and acid-base status, his _____ (respiratory, metabolic) _____ (acidosis, alkalosis) is caused by a _____ (gain, loss) of base.

46. Mr. Lawson's metabolic acid-base imbalance (question #45) is present with a(n) _____ (normal, abnormal) anion gap. This is called _____ (hyperchloremia, hypochloremia) metabolic _____ (acidosis, alkalosis) because the loss of base is related to an _____ (excessive, inadequate) chloride ions in the plasma.

47. Ms. Johnson, a patient in the kidney dialysis unit, has the following blood gas and electrolyte results: pH = 7.17, $PaCO_2$ = 31 mm Hg, HCO_3^- = 11 mEq/L, Na^+ = 136 mEq/L; Cl^- 99 mEq/L. Based on her anion gap and acid-base status, her _____ (respiratory, metabolic) _____ (acidosis, alkalosis) is caused by a _____ (gain, loss) of fixed acid.

48. Ms. Johnson's condition (question #47) shows metabolic _____ (acidosis, alkalosis) with a(n) _____ (increased, normal, decreased) anion gap. This condition may be produced by the body as seen in _____ (renal failure, alcohol poisoning), or added from an external source as seen in _____ (renal failure, alcohol poisoning).

49. In patients with adequate lung function, respiratory compensation of metabolic acidosis usually takes place in the form of _____ (hyperventilation, hypoventilation).

50. During mechanical ventilation, respiratory compensation may occur due to metabolic acidosis. The ventilator rate can be reduced when hyperventilation is documented by a low $PaCO_2$.

    (TRUE/FALSE)

51. Severe K^+ depletion can lead to metabolic _____ (acidosis, alkalosis) and compensatory _____ (hyperventilation, hypoventilation).

ARTERIAL BLOOD GASES

52 to 54. Fill in the normal ranges of the blood gas parameters.

MONITORING FUNCTION	PARAMETER	NORMAL (P_B 760 mm Hg)
52. Gas Exchange	$PaCO_2$	_____ to _____ mm Hg
53. Oxygenation	PaO_2	_____ to _____ mm Hg
54. Acid-Base	pH	_____ to _____

55. Direct measurement of the arterial _____ (pH, PaO_2, $PaCO_2$) via arterial puncture or indwelling catheter is the most accurate method of assessing a patient's ventilatory status.

56. Hypoventilation and respiratory _____ (acidosis, alkalosis) are present when the $PaCO_2$ is _____ (increased, decreased) with a concurrent decrease in pH. This condition may be corrected by _____ (increasing, decreasing) the rate or tidal volume on the ventilator.

57. Hyperventilation and respiratory _____ (acidosis, alkalosis) are present when the $PaCO_2$ is _____ (increased, decreased) with a concurrent increase in pH. This condition is usually be corrected by _____ (increasing, decreasing) the rate on the ventilator.

58. Tidal volume or rate control on the ventilator may be used to correct metabolic acid-base abnormalities during mechanical ventilation.

    (TRUE/FALSE)

59. Patients with depressed central respiratory drive, elevated V_D/V_T, diminished compliance, or respiratory muscle weakness may develop _____ (excessive renal compensation, respiratory muscle fatigue) and _____ (renal failure, ventilatory failure).

60. A(n) _____ (increased, decreased) PaO2, a(n) _____ (increased, decreased) $P(A-a)O_2$, or a(n) _____ (increased, decreased) PaO_2/PAO^2 can be used as an indicator of tissue hypoxia.

61. Ms. Zadori, an 36-year-old asthmatic patient, has an arterial PO_2 of 48 mm Hg while breathing room air. Her oxygenation status can be interpreted as _____ (mild, moderate, severe) hypoxemia.

62. A 59-year-old patient has a calculated $P(A-a)O_2$ of 36 mm Hg while breathing room air. The patient's oxygenation status is interpreted as _____ (normal, hypoxemia) since the normal $P(A-a)O_2$ for a 59-year-old should be _____ (more than 36 mm Hg, less than 24 mm Hg).

63. Mr. Protschka, a 55-year-old postoperative patient, has a $P(A-a)O_2$ of 353 mm Hg while breathing 100% oxygen. His estimated intrapulmonary shunt is:
    A. 10%.
    B. 12%.
    C. 14%.
    D. 16%.

64. The normal PaO_2/PAO_2 ratio should be greater than _____ on an F_IO_2 of 30% or higher. A PaO_2/PAO_2 ratio of 60% is indicative of a _____ (hyperoxic, normal oxygenation, hypoxic) state.

65. When hypoxemia is caused by acute hypoventilation, immediate treatment with oxygen should be sufficient.

    (TRUE/FALSE).

    Explain why or why not.

    _____

66. Hypoxemia caused by ventilation/perfusion (V/Q) mismatch is characterized by a _____ (high, normal or low) $PaCO_2$ and it usually responds _____ (well, poorly) to moderate level of supplemental oxygen.

67. Hypoxemia caused by intrapulmonary shunting is characterized by a _____ (high, normal or low) $PaCO_2$ and it usually shows _____ (excellent, good, poor) response to moderate level of supplemental oxygen.

68. Refractory hypoxemia (hypoxemia that does not respond to oxygen therapy alone) should be treated with oxygen therapy and:
    A. mechanical ventilation.
    B. pressure support.
    C. hyperbaric oxygen therapy.
    D. positive end-expiratory pressure.

69. _____ is a mechanism of gas diffusion abnormalities that may lead to hypoxemia.
    A. High oxygen pressure gradient
    B. Decreased alveolar-capillary thickness
    C. Decreased alveolar surface area
    D. High F_IO_2

70 to 72. Match the types of gas diffusion defects with the examples. Use each answer only once.

DIFFUSION DEFECT	EXAMPLE
70. Low alveolar-arterial oxygen tension gradient	A. Emphysema
71. Increased alveolar-capillary membrane thickness	B. High altitude
72. Decreased alveolar surface area	C. Pulmonary edema

OXYGEN SATURATION MONITORING

73. In comparison to pulse oximetry oxygen saturation (SpO_2), arterial oxygen saturation (SaO_2) is:
    A. less accurate.
    B. a more invasive measurement.
    C. more expensive to measure.
    D. suitable for adults only.

74. Pulse oximetry may be used to perform all of the following *except*:
    A. intermittent measurement of SpO_2.
    B. continuous monitoring of SpO_2.
    C. measurement of heart rate.
    D. measurement of PaO_2.

75. The heart rate measurement on the oximeter is normally faster than the heart rate obtained by a cardiac monitor.

    (TRUE/FALSE)

76. SpO_2 is very accurate and it correlates with SaO_2 when the arterial oxygen saturation is greater than 75% or PaO_2 greater than 50 mm Hg.

    (TRUE/FALSE)

77. SpO_2 measurements are useful in all of the following clinical applications *except*:
    A. assessment of ventilatory status.
    B. weaning from mechanical ventilation.
    C. adjustment of F_IO_2.
    D. reduction of arterial punctures.

78. The recent blood gas report of a patient shows: pH = 7.38, $PaCO_2$ = 46 mm Hg, PaO_2 = 43 mm Hg, SaO_2 = 78%. Since the patient does not show signs of respiratory distress or hypoxia, you would initially verify the accuracy of this blood gas report by:

    A. performing another arterial puncture.

    B. measuring the electrolyte level.

    C. measuring the SpO_2.

    D. recommending a stat chest radiograph.

79. The blood gas and pulse oximetry measurements for a postoperative patient are: pH = 7.37, $PaCO_2$ = 47 mm Hg, PaO_2 = 41 mm Hg, SaO_2 = 78%, SpO_2 = 96%. What is the interpretation of these results?

    A. venous blood gas sample

    B. moderate hypoxemia

    C. hypoventilation

    D. compensated respiratory acidosis

80. SpO_2 and SaO_2 correlate extremely well when the SaO_2 is 95% or greater.

    (TRUE/FALSE)

81. SpO_2 becomes less accurate as SaO_2 _____ (increases, decreases) and it _____ (overestimates, underestimates) a patient's oxygenation status at _____ (high, low) SaO_2 levels.

82. Sunlight, fluorescent light, nail polish (primarily blue, green, and black), nail coverings, and intravascular dyes may produce a falsely _____ (high, low) SpO_2 reading.

83. Low perfusion states and presence of dyshemoglobins may lead to SpO_2 measurements that are _____ (higher, lower) than the actual SaO_2.

84. Mr. King, a patient who was found in a burning house, is reported to have SpO_2 measurements in the upper 90's while breathing spontaneously on 5 L/min of oxygen via a simple mask. Upon his transfer from the ambulance to emergency room, you would immediately perform all of the following *except*:

    A. change to a non-rebreathing mask.

    B. change to 15 L/min oxygen.

    C. obtain carboxyhemoglobin measurement.

    D. start aerosol therapy with albuterol and saline.

END-TIDAL CARBON DIOXIDE MONITORING

85. End-tidal carbon dioxide monitoring is done to monitor a patient's _____ (circulatory, oxygenation, ventilatory) status.

86. Capnography is a measurement of the partial pressure of _____ (oxygen, carbon monoxide, carbon dioxide) during _____ (the inspiratory phase, the expiratory phase, a complete respiratory cycle).

87. When the sample is collected at the end of inspiration, it is called end-tidal partial pressure of carbon dioxide ($PetCO_2$).

    (TRUE/FALSE)

88. The major advantage of mainstream $PetCO_2$ analyzer and the attachments is its _____ (fast response time, light weight, low dead space volume).

89. The major advantage of sidestream $PetCO_2$ analyzer and the attachments is its _____ (high deadspace volume, ease of handling, cleanliness).

90. In analyzing a complete capnography waveform, at beginning-exhalation the $PECO_2$ measurement is near _____ (0%, 5%, 15%, 30%) signifying the anatomic dead space volume exiting the airways.

91. The end-tidal PCO_2 ($PetCO_2$) on a complete capnography waveform is the reading taken at the _____ (first, middle, last) part of the waveform at the _____ (beginning, end) of the alveolar plateau.

92. The capnogram can be useful in evaluating or managing all of the following conditions *except*:
    A. esophageal intubation.
    B. endotracheal tube cuff leaks.
    C. hypocapnic management of head trauma.
    D. oxygenation status.

93. The normal gradient between $PaCO_2$ and $PetCO_2$ is about _____ (2, 5, 10) mm Hg in healthy individuals and _____ (2, 5, 10) mm Hg in critically ill patients.

94 to 96. Certain clinical conditions can increase the $P(a\text{-}et)CO_2$ gradient. Match the clinical conditions with the factors affecting the $P(a\text{-}et)CO_2$ gradient.

CLINICAL CONDITION	FACTORS
94. Ventilation	A. During coronary artery bypass surgery
95. Perfusion	B. Increased dead space ventilation
96. Temperature	C. Decreased cardiac output

97. A low cost, disposable, plastic CO_2 (pH) sensitive device may be used as an attachment to the endotracheal tube to assess _____ (hypoventilation, hypoxia, esophageal intubation).

98. Dead space ventilation (e.g., pulmonary embolism) *or* improvement of ventilation causes a(n) _____ (increase, decrease) of $PetCO_2$.

99. Explain why the ventilator rate should *not* be decreased when a decrease in $PetCO_2$ is due to dead space ventilation.

_____

_____

100. Hypotension and high intrathoracic pressure secondary to mechanical ventilation may cause a(n) _____ (increase, decrease) in $PetCO_2$. Under these conditions, the ventilator rate _____ (should, should not) be reduced because this $PetCO_2$ change _____ (does, does not) imply that ventilation has improved.

TRANSCUTANEOUS BLOOD GAS MEASUREMENT

101. Transcutaneous blood gas monitoring involves use of a miniature Clark electrode for the _____ (PO_2, PCO_2, pH) measurement and a Severinghaus electrode for the _____ (PO_2, PCO_2, pH) measurement.

102. Transcutaneous blood gas monitoring involves placement of the electrode _____ (over the artery, over the vein, on the skin). A heating coil is used in the electrode to _____ (increase, decrease) the permeability of the epidermis thus facilitating diffusion of gas from the underlying capillaries to the electrode.

103. Transcutaneous blood gas monitoring has been used extensively in neonates and adults.

    (TRUE/FALSE)

104. In neonates, the $PtcO_2$ closely approximates the PaO_2. In adults, the $PtcO_2$ measures _____ (higher, lower) than the actual PO_2 due to _____.

105. List three conditions that may affect the accuracy of a $PtcO_2$ electrode.

    _____

106. $PtcO_2$ is a better predictor of PaO_2 when the PaO_2 is _____ (above, below) 80 mm Hg and it becomes less accurate when the PaO_2 is _____ (greater, less) than 80 mm Hg.

107. Hypothermia, increase in skin thickness, decrease in cardiac output may cause a disproportionate _____ (rise, fall) in the $PtcO_2$ readings.

108. One disadvantage of transcutaneous monitors is the need for site changes every _____ (1 to 2, 3 to 4, 4 to 6) hours to prevent damage of skin due to the _____ (heating element, tape on the electrode, chemical on the adhesive disc).

109. $PtcCO_2$ monitoring is done to provide continuous _____ (oxygenation, ventilatory) assessment. The $PtcCO_2$ is measured by heating the underlying skin to about _____ (37, 42, 47)°C to facilitate CO_2 diffusion across the skin to the CO_2 electrode.

110. The $PtcCO_2$ values are usually _____ (higher, lower) than the $PaCO_2$ values. This is due to _____ (increased, decreased) CO_2 production as the underlying tissues are heated.

111. During shock or low perfusion states, the $PtcCO_2$ becomes _____ (higher, lower) than the actual $PaCO_2$ due to _____ (increased, decreased) accumulation of CO_2 in the tissues.

CHAPTER TEN

HEMODYNAMIC WAVEFORM ANALYSIS

HEMODYNAMIC MONITORING

1. Preload is a measurement that reflects the volume of blood _____ (entering, remaining in, leaving) a heart ventricle, and is expressed in a pressure unit of cm H_2O or mm Hg.

2. Since the central venous drainage returns to the pulmonary circulation via the _____ (left, right) heart, the central venous pressure is known as the _____ (left, right) ventricular _____ (preload, afterload).

3. Central venous pressure is measured by a _____ catheter.

4. Afterload is a measurement that reflects the volume of blood _____ (entering, remaining in, leaving) a heart ventricle, also expressed in a pressure unit of cm H_2O or mm Hg.

5. Since the pulmonary arteries receive the blood from the _____ (left, right) heart, pulmonary artery pressure is called the _____ (left, right) ventricular _____ (preload, afterload).

6. Pulmonary artery pressure is measured by a _____ catheter.

7. The left ventricular preload is not simply the pulmonary artery pressure. It is measured by wedging the pulmonary artery with an inflated balloon located at the tip of the pulmonary artery catheter. A small branch of the pulmonary artery is wedged in order to _____ (enhance, stop) the blood flow. The pressure thus obtained accurately reflects the volume status _____ (with, without) the effects of blood flow and vascular resistance.

8. Measurement of hemodynamic pressures is based upon the principle that liquids are _____ (compressible, non-compressible) and that pressures at any given point within a liquid are transmitted _____ (equally, unevenly).

9. When a closed system is filled with liquid, the pressure exerted at one point can be measured accurately at any other point on the same level.

(TRUE/FALSE)

10. Complete hemodynamic monitoring is done by using three catheters. Name these three catheters.

    _____

11. To minimize the effects of gravity, the transducer, catheter, and measurement site should be at the same level. A higher reading may be obtained if the transducer and catheter are located _____ (higher, lower) than the measurement site.

12. Hazards and complications of hemodynamic monitoring include all of the following *except*:

    A. fluid overload.

    B. infection.

    C. dysrhythmia.

    D. bleeding.

13. A PaO_2 measurement of 100 mm Hg in the United States is equal to _____ (1.33, 13.3, 100, 133) pKa in other countries using the Systeme International (SI) units.

14. Three different catheters are used in hemodynamic monitoring: The arterial catheter is placed in a _____ (pulmonary, systemic) artery. The central venous catheter is placed in the superior vena cava or _____ (right, left atrium). The pulmonary artery (Swan-Ganz) catheter is placed in a _____ (pulmonary, systemic) artery.

ARTERIAL CATHETER

15. Name four common arteries for placement of an arterial catheter.

    _____

16. Among the arteries accessible for arterial catheter insertion, the _____ (radial, brachial, femoral) artery is the first choice because collateral circulation to the hand is also provided by the _____ artery.

17. An arterial catheter can be used to gather all of the following information *except*:

    A. central venous pressure.

    B. systolic pressure.

    C. diastolic pressure.

    D. arterial blood gases.

18. The characteristic dicrotic notch on an arterial pressure waveform is caused by the _____ (opening, closure) of the _____ (aortic, pulmonic, mitral, tricuspid) valve during _____ (contraction, relaxation) of the ventricles.

19. Upon reviewing a patient's vital signs, you notice that the systemic systolic and diastolic pressures are 100/70 mm Hg. Are they within the normal range? What is the calculated mean arterial pressure?

    A. Yes; 60 mm Hg

    B. Yes; 80 mm Hg

    C. No; 60 mm Hg

    D. No; 80 mm Hg

20. How is the mean arterial pressure used to assess the adequacy of tissue perfusion?

_____

21. Since arterial pressure is the _____ (sum, difference, product) of blood flow and vascular resistance, an increase of cardiac output *or* vasoconstriction would _____ (increase, decrease) the arterial pressure. A decrease of cardiac output *or* vasodilation would _____ (increase, decrease) the arterial pressure.

22. Pulse pressure is the difference between arterial systolic and diastolic pressure as shown below.
    A. Pulse pressure = $P_{SYSTOLIC} + P_{DIASTOLIC}$
    B. Pulse pressure = $P_{SYSTOLIC} - P_{DIASTOLIC}$
    C. Pulse pressure = $P_{SYSTOLIC} \times P_{DIASTOLIC}$
    D. Pulse pressure = $P_{SYSTOLIC} / P_{DIASTOLIC}$

23. A high systolic pressure ($P_{SYSTOLIC}$) *or* a low diastolic pressure ($P_{DIASTOLIC}$) would _____ (increase, decrease) the pulse pressure.

24. A low systolic pressure ($P_{SYSTOLIC}$) *or* a high diastolic pressure ($P_{DIASTOLIC}$) would _____ (increase, decrease) the pulse pressure.

25. Pulse pressure is *least* affected by a patient's changing:
    A. stroke volume.
    B. blood vessel compliance.
    C. heart rate.
    D. spontaneous tidal volume.

26. High pulse pressure may reflect _____ (increased, decreased) stroke volume, _____ (increased, decreased) blood vessel compliance, or _____ (increased, decreased) heart rate.

27. Low pulse pressure may reflect _____ (increased, decreased) stroke volume, _____ (increased, decreased) blood vessel compliance, or _____ (increased, decreased) heart rate.

28 to 32. Match the factors affecting the arterial catheter with the related problems. Use each answer only once.

FACTORS	PROBLEM
28. Air bubbles in tubing Loose tubing connections	A. Measurement lower than actual
	B. Back-up of blood in the tubing
29. Transducer and catheter placed higher than measurement site	C. Inaccurate reading Signal interference
30. Transducer and catheter placed lower than measurement site	D. Dampened pressure signal
	E. Measurement higher than actual
31. Inadequate pressure applied to the heparin solution bag	
32. Blood clot at catheter tip Catheter tip blocked by wall of artery	

CENTRAL VENOUS CATHETER

33. The central venous pressure (CVP) is monitored through a central venous catheter placed either in the _____ (superior, inferior) vena cava near the _____ (left, right) atrium or in the _____ (left, right) atrium.

34. CVP measures the filling pressures in the _____ (left, right) heart. Therefore it is helpful in assessing the fluid status of the _____ (systemic, pulmonary) circulation.

35. CVP may also be used to assess the _____ (left, right) heart function but it is often late to reflect changes in the _____ (left, right) heart.

36. The central venous catheter can also be used to collect _____ (venous, mixed venous, arterial) blood samples and for administration of medications and fluids.

37. The central venous catheter is commonly inserted through the _____ vein or the _____ vein.

38 to 42. In reference to Figure 10-3 of the textbook *Clinical Application of Mechanical Ventilation*, match the waves and downslopes of a central venous (right atrial) pressure tracing with the events during a cardiac contraction.

WAVE OR DOWNSLOPE	EVENT
38. Upstroke *a* wave	A. closure of the tricuspid valve during systole
39. *c* wave	B. right ventricular contraction
40. *x* downslope	C. relaxation of ventricle
41. *v* wave	D. right atrial contraction
42. *y* downslope	E. relaxation of right atrium

43. Changes in the hemodynamic status of the heart will cause changes to certain components of the right atrial tracing, particularly the *a* and *v* waves.

    (TRUE/FALSE)

44. The *a* wave on the right atrial waveform may be _____ (elevated, depressed, absent) when the resistance to *right* ventricular filling is increased as in _____ (mitral, tricuspid) valve stenosis. The *a* wave may be _____ (elevated, depressed, absent) if the atrial activity is absent or extremely weak.

45. Reflux of blood into the right atrium during contraction due to an incompetent triscupid valve will cause a(n) _____ (elevated, depressed, absent) *v* wave.

46. _____ (Elevation, Depression, Absence) of *a* and *v* waves may be seen in conditions such as cardiac tamponade, volume overload, or left ventricular failure.

47. The normal range of CVP measured in the superior vena cava is from _____ to _____ mm Hg. When the measurement is taken in the right atrium, the normal value ranges from _____ to _____ mm Hg, slightly _____ (higher, lower) than the reading taken in the vena cava.

48. Since venous return (systemic to pulmonary circulation) is determined by the pressure gradient between the mean arterial pressure and CVP, an increased CVP leads to a _____ (larger, smaller) pressure gradient and a _____ (higher, lower) blood return to the right heart.

49. Since positive pressure ventilation increases the CVP, it leads to a(n) _____ (increased, decreased) venous return and a _____ (higher, lower) cardiac output.

50. The CVP may be decreased in all of the following clinical conditions *except*:
    A. right ventricular failure.
    B. severe blood loss.
    C. fluid depletion.
    D. shock.

51. The CVP may be increased in all of the following clinical conditions *except*:
    A. positive pressure ventilation.
    B. vasodilation.
    C. pulmonary hypertension.
    D. fluid overload.

PULMONARY ARTERY CATHETER

52. The pulmonary artery (Swan-Ganz) catheter is a flow directed, balloon-tipped catheter and with proper accessories it can measure all of the following *except*:
    A. cardiac output.
    B. mixed venous oxygen saturation.
    C. arterial oxygen saturation.
    D. pulmonary capillary wedge pressure.

53. The pulmonary artery catheter is usually inserted into either the _____ or _____ vein. From there it is advanced to the superior vena cava and _____ (left, right) atrium. The balloon is then inflated and the blood flow moves the catheter through the _____ (left, right) ventricle and into the _____ (systemic, pulmonary) artery where it will eventually "wedge" in a smaller branch of the artery.

54. After successful placement of the pulmonary artery catheter, the balloon is kept _____ (inflated, deflated) and the catheter stabilized in place. The balloon is _____ (inflated, deflated) only when the pulmonary capillary wedge pressure is being taken.

55. List the three components of a typical pulmonary arterial pressure waveform.

    _____

56. The characteristic dicrotic notch on the PAP waveform reflects _____ (opening, closure) of the pulmonic valve at the end of contraction and prior to the refilling of ventricles.

57. The systolic component of the pulmonary artery pressure waveform may be increased in conditions in which the pulmonary vascular resistance or pulmonary blood flow is _____ (increased, decreased).

58. Pulmonary arterial pressure (PAP) is measured when the pulmonary artery (Swan-Ganz) catheter is inside the pulmonary artery with the balloon _____ (inflated, deflated).

59. The normal systolic PAP is about _____ (5 mm Hg higher than, the same as, 5 mm Hg lower than) the right ventricular systolic pressure.

60. The normal systolic PAP ranges from _____ to _____ mm Hg and the normal diastolic PAP range is from _____ to _____ mm Hg.

61. Positive end-expiratory pressure (PEEP) can _____ (increase, decrease) the PAP because overdistension of the alveoli compresses the surrounding capillaries and _____ (raises, lowers) the capillary and arterial pressures.

62. Increase of pulmonary vascular resistance or pulmonary blood flow can also lead to a(n) _____ (increased, decreased) PAP because the pressure measurement is _____ (directly, inversely) related to the resistance and blood flow.

63. Left ventricular failure and mitral valve disease may cause a(n) _____ (increased, decreased) PAP because obstruction or backup of blood flow in the left heart leads to congestion in the pulmonary circulation.

64. The PAP may be decreased in conditions of _____ (hypervolemia, hypovolemia) or use of mechanical ventilation.

65. When positive pressure ventilation is used on patients who have unstable hemodynamic status, it may lead to a depressed cardiac output, venous return, pulmonary circulating volume, and PAP.

    (TRUE/FALSE)

66. Positive pressure ventilation (without PEEP) may cause a decrease of PAP due to the resultant _____ (increased, decreased) venous return, _____ (higher, lower) right ventricular output, and _____ (higher, lower) blood volume (pressure) in the pulmonary arteries.

67. In the absence of compensation by increasing the heart rate, a decrease of right and left ventricular stroke volume generally leads to a(n) _____ (increased, decreased) cardiac output.

68. Complete the table below.

    Positive pressure ventilation (without PEEP)

    ↓

    _____ (Increase, Decrease) in intrathoracic pressure

    ↓

    _____ (Increase, Decrease) in venous return

    ↓

    _____ (Higher, Lower) right ventricular output

    ↓

    _____ (Higher, Lower) blood volume (pressure) in the pulmonary artery

69. The pulmonary artery catheter may also be used to measure the pulmonary capillary wedge pressure (PCWP) by slowly _____ (inflating, deflating) the balloon until the wedged pressure waveform is seen. Proper inflation of the balloon usually requires no more than _____ (1, 3, 5) cc of air. The balloon is _____ (inflated, deflated) as soon as the reading of PCWP is made.

70 to 74. In reference to Figure 10-9 of the textbook *Clinical Application of Mechanical Ventilation*, match the waves and downslopes of a pulmonary capillary wedge pressure tracing with the events during a cardiac contraction.

WAVE OR DOWNSLOPE	EVENT
70. Upstroke *a* wave	A. left ventricular contraction
71. *c* wave	B. closure of the mitral valve during systole
72. *x* downslope	C. relaxation of left atrium
73. *v* wave	D. left atrial contraction
74. *y* downslope	E. relaxation of ventricle

75. A(n) _____ (increase, decrease) of PCWP measurements are often observed in conditions where partial obstruction or excessive blood flow is present in the left heart.

76. The *a* wave of the PCWP waveform may be increased in conditions leading to _____ (higher, lower) resistance to left ventricular filling as in _____ (mitral valve, tricuspid) stenosis.

77. The *v* wave of the PCWP waveform may be _____ (increased, decreased) due to regurgitation (backward flow) of blood from the left ventricle to the left atrium through the incompetent mitral valve.

78. The normal PCWP range is from _____ to _____ mm Hg.

79. The PCWP may be _____ (increased, decreased) during positive pressure ventilation or PEEP due to overdistension of the alveoli or compression of the surrounding capillaries.

80. The PCWP may be _____ (increased, decreased) during left ventricular failure because of backup of blood flow in the left heart and pulmonary circulation.

81. The PCWP measurement may be used to distinguish cardiogenic and noncardiogenic pulmonary edema. In pulmonary edema that is caused by left ventricular failure, the PCWP is usually _____ (elevated, normal, decreased).

82. When pulmonary edema occurs with a(n) _____ (elevated, normal, decreased) PCWP, it is probably due to an increase of the capillary permeability as seen in ARDS.

83. A pulmonary artery catheter has just been inserted and the presence of artifacts make identification of the PCWP tracing difficult. The physician asks you to evaluate whether the catheter is properly wedged. You would choose any of the following methods *except*:
    A. postcapillary-mixed venous PO_2 gradient.
    B. postcapillary-mixed venous O_2 saturation gradient.
    C. PAP systolic-PCWP gradient.
    D. PAP diastolic-PCWP gradient.

84. Under normal conditions, the average wedge pressure is about 1 to 4 mm Hg _____ (higher, lower) than the PAP _____ (systolic, diastolic) value.

85. Since a properly wedged catheter does not allow mixing of shunted venous blood with the postcapillary blood, the PO_2 of a blood gas sample from the distal opening of a properly wedged catheter should be at least 19 mm Hg _____ (higher, lower) than that obtained from a systemic artery. The PCO_2 should be at least 11 mm Hg _____ (higher, lower).

86. For the same reason that a properly wedged pulmonary artery catheter does not allow mixing of venous blood, the oxygen saturation value of a properly wedged catheter should be about 20% _____ (higher, lower) than the oxygen saturation recorded with the balloon deflated.

87. Another important value of the pulmonary artery catheter is its ability to _____ (estimate, measure) cardiac output by the thermodilution technique.

88. The normal cardiac output for an adult is from _____ to _____ L/min.

89. Cardiac index is used to assess a person's measured cardiac output in reference to the patient's _____ (tidal volume, oxygen consumption, body size) and the normal cardiac index ranges from 2.5 to 3.5 L/min/m^2.

SUMMARY OF PRELOADS AND AFTERLOADS

90. Measurements obtained with a systemic arterial catheter reflect the _____ (left, right) ventricular _____ (preload, afterload). For example, the arterial pressure is _____ (increased, decreased) in systemic hypertension or fluid overload.

91. Measurements obtained with a central venous catheter reflect the _____ (left, right) ventricular _____ (preload, afterload). For example, the central venous pressure is _____ (increased, decreased) in systemic hypotension or hypovolemia.

92. Measurements obtained with a pulmonary artery catheter (with the balloon deflated) reflect the _____ (left, right) ventricular _____ (preload, afterload). For example, the pulmonary artery pressure is _____ (increased, decreased) in pulmonary hypertension or blood flow obstruction in the left heart.

93. Measurements obtained with a pulmonary artery catheter (with the balloon inflated) reflect the _____ (left, right) ventricular _____ (preload, afterload). For example, the pulmonary capillary wedge pressure is _____ (increased, decreased) in severe hypotension or dehydration.

CALCULATED HEMODYNAMIC VALUES

94. The stroke volume (S.V.) is calculated by which of the following equations? [C.O. = cardiac output, HR = heart rate, BSA = body surface area]
    A. S.V. = C.O. × HR
    B. S.V. = C.O. / HR
    C. S.V. = C.O. × BSA
    D. S.V. = C.O. / BSA

95. Explain how changes of contractility, preload, and afterload would affect the stroke volume.

_____

_____

_____

96. Oxygen consumption (VO$_2$) may be calculated by which of the following equations? [Q$_T$ = total perfusion (cardiac output), C(a-v)O$_2$ = arterial-mixed venous oxygen content difference, BSA = body surface area]
    A. $VO_2 = Q_T \times BSA$
    B. $VO_2 = Q_T / BSA$
    C. $VO_2 = Q_T \times C(a\text{-}v)O_2$
    D. $VO_2 = Q_T / C(a\text{-}v)O_2$

97. The pulmonary vascular resistance (PVR) measures the vascular resistance to blood flow in the _____ (systemic, pulmonary) circulation and it may be elevated in pulmonary _____ (hypertension, hypotension).

98. The systemic vascular resistance (SVR) measures the vascular resistance to blood flow in the _____ (systemic, pulmonary) circulation and it may be elevated in fluid _____ (overload, depletion).

MONITORING OF MIXED VENOUS OXYGEN SATURATION

99. The normal SvO$_2$ is about _____ %. SvO$_2$ of less than _____ % is indicative of hypoxemia or hypoxia.

100 to 102. Some clinical conditions may decrease the SvO$_2$ measurements. Match the conditions with the examples. Use *only three* of the answers provided.

CONDITIONS	EXAMPLES
100. Poor oxygen supply	A. Severe and prolonged hypoxia
101. Excessive oxygen demand	B. Decreased cardiac output
102. Depletion of venous oxygen reserve	C. Cyanide poisoning
	D. Decreased metabolic rate
	E. Increased metabolic rate

103 to 105. Some clinical conditions may increase the SvO$_2$ measurements. Match the conditions with the examples. Use *only three* of the answers provided.

CONDITIONS	EXAMPLES
103. Technical problem	A. Sepsis
104. Impaired oxygen utilization	B. Increased physical activity
105. Decrease of oxygen demand	C. Hypothermia
	D. Increased cardiac output
	E. Improperly wedged catheter

CHAPTER ELEVEN

BASIC VENTILATOR WAVEFORM ANALYSIS

FLOW WAVES USED FOR POSITIVE PRESSURE VENTILATION

1. The _____ (square and descending, accelerating and sine) flow waveforms are not used for positive pressure ventilation because the initial flow rate is _____ (too high, not sufficient) for most patients.

2. Accelerating and sine waveforms may be appropriate for _____ (assist, intermittent mandatory ventilation, control, pressure support, pressure control, inverse ratio) mode of mechanical ventilation.

EFFECTS OF CONSTANT FLOW DURING VOLUME-CONTROLLED VENTILATION

3. In flow and pressure waveforms, _____ (flow or pressure measurement, time in seconds) is displayed along the *y* or vertical axis.

4. The area under a flow waveform can be used to estimate the _____ (pressure setting, tidal volume, peak flow, mean airway pressure).

5. Under normal conditions, the area enclosed under the expiratory flow waveform should be _____ (greater than, equal to, less than) the area under the inspiratory flow waveform.

6. In mechanical ventilation, _____ (obstruction, gas leak, tension pneumothorax) may be present if the expiratory volume is less than the inspiratory volume.

7. In assist/control mode of mechanical ventilation, the I:E ratio is _____ (constant, variable). This is because an assist breath that comes earlier than expected would _____ (prolong, shorten) the _____ (inspiratory, expiratory) time of the previous breath.

8. On a pressure waveform, _____ (pressure support, PIP, PEEP) is present when the end-expiratory pressure rests above 0 cm H_2O.

SPONTANEOUS VENTILATION DURING MECHANICAL VENTILATION

9. On the pressure waveform, assist effort is present when the trigger pressure reaches the _____ (tidal volume, sensitivity, pressure limit, peak flow).

10. _____ (PEEP, CPAP, Pressure support ventilation) describes a pressure waveform in which there are no mechanical breaths and the airway pressure is above 0 cm H_2O.

EFFECTS OF FLOW, CIRCUIT AND LUNG CHARACTERISTICS ON PRESSURE-TIME WAVEFORMS

11. An increase in _____ (total compliance, airflow resistance) would result in an unchanged P_{ALV} but increased PIP and P_{TA}.

12. A decrease in _____ (total compliance, airflow resistance) would result in an unchanged P_{TA} but increased PIP and P_{ALV}.

EFFECTS OF DECELERATING FLOW DURING VOLUME-CONTROLLED VENTILATION

13. When the flow waveform selection is changed from square to decelerating during _____ (pressure limited, time limited, flow limited), same volume can only be maintained if the *peak flow* of the decelerating pattern is increased.

14. When the flow waveform selection is changed from square to decelerating during _____ (pressure limited, time limited, flow limited), same volume can only be maintained if the *inspiratory time* of the decelerating pattern is increased.

15. With time limited ventilation, the decelerating flow creates a _____ (higher, lower) *initial* peak flow and _____ (higher, lower) initial flow resistive pressure (P_{TA}) than that created by the square flow.

16. With flow limited ventilation, the initial flow resistive pressure (P_{TA}) is the same for the _____ (sine and accelerating, square and decelerating) flow waves.

17. In square and decelerating flow ventilation, the rise in alveolar pressure (P_{ALV}) is directly related to the _____ (tidal volume, compliance, resistance) and inversely related to _____ (tidal volume, compliance, resistance).

18. At constant Ti, a decreased flow leads to _____ (higher, lower) V_T, P_{TA}, and P_{ALV}.

19. A higher end flow leads to a _____ (larger, smaller) V_T and it does not affect the P_{TA} and P_{ALV}.

20. When peak flow is kept unchanged, V_T, Ti and P_{ALV} are _____ (directly, inversely) related.

WAVEFORMS DEVELOPED DURING PRESSURE-LIMITED VENTILATION

21. In pressure control ventilation, _____, _____, _____ are typically set by the operator.

22. In pressure control ventilation, the flow level and V_T are dependent on the _____.

23. In _____ (pressure support, inverse ratio pressure control) ventilation, the patients are usually sedated and paralyzed in order to prevent dyssynchrony with the ventilator.

PRESSURE SUPPORT AND SPONTANEOUS MODES OF VENTILATION

24. In pressure support ventilation, the patient controls the _____.

EFFECTS OF LUNG CHARACTERISTICS ON PRESSURE-LIMITED WAVEFORMS

25. During pressure-limited ventilation, an increased airflow resistance or a decreased compliance would reduce the delivered flow and _____.

USING WAVEFORMS FOR PATIENT AND VENTILATOR-SYSTEM ASSESSMENT

26. Tachypnea, agitation, accessory muscle usage, active expiration, muscle fatigue, and respiratory failure are signs of _____.

27. On a flow waveform, failure of the expiratory flow to return to baseline is indicative of incomplete _____ (inspiration, expiration) and this condition may lead to _____ (hyperventilation, gas trapping).

USING THE EXPIRATORY FLOW AND PRESSURE WAVES AS DIAGNOSTIC TOOLS

28. Excessive airway resistance during mechanical ventilation would cause a(n) _____ (increased, decreased) expiratory flow and a(n) _____ (increased, decreased) expiratory time.

29. A decreased C_{LT} leads to a higher expiratory peak flow, a _____ (higher, lower) PIP and a _____ (longer, shorter) expiratory time.

TROUBLESHOOTING VENTILATOR MALFUNCTION

30. A delay of positive pressure waveform (i.e., lack of ventilator response) in spite of a normal negative pressure waveform (i.e., good patient effort) is indicative of:
    A. inadequate line pressure.
    B. ventilator malfunction.
    C. dysfunction of the inspiratory valve or sensitivity setting.
    D. electrical malfunction.

31. Failure of the expiratory flow to return to the zero baseline is indicative of:
    A. gas leak.
    B. airflow obstruction.
    C. power failure.
    D. high lung compliance.

32. Auto-triggering and fast mechanical breaths may develop when _____ (airflow obstruction, circuit leak) occurs during mechanical ventilation with PEEP. This is because the pressure in the circuit _____ (rises to the PEEP level, drops to the sensitivity setting below the PEEP level).

PRESSURE-VOLUME AND FLOW-VOLUME CURVES OR LOOPS

33. (Refer to Figure 11-38 in textbook.) The difference between P_{ALV} and P_{AO} is _____ (PEEP, P_{TA}, PIP, C_{LT}).

34. (Refer to Figure 11-38 in textbook.) On a pressure-volume curve, a linear increase in P_{ALV} with increases in volume is the characteristic of a stable _____ (PIP, PEEP, C_{LT}).

35. On a pressure-volume curve (PVC), a reduction in C_{LT} causes the PVC to move down and to the _____ (left, right).

36. On a pressure-volume curve, a reduction in C_{LT} will not change the P_{TA} because the gradient between _____ remains the same. (See Figure 11-39 in textbook.)
    A. P_{TA} and P_{AO}
    B. P_{AO} and P_{ALV}
    C. P_{IP} and P_{AO}
    D. PIP and P_{ALV}

37. On a pressure-volume curve, an increase in resistance would not affect the _____ while the _____ are increased. (See Figure 11-40.)
    A. P_{ALV}; P_{TA} and PIP
    B. P_{ALV}; P_{TA}, PIP and P_{AO}
    C. P_{TA}; PIP and P_{AO}
    D. P_{TA}; PAO, PIP and P_{ALV}

38. The initial point of inflection (Ipi) occurs when alveoli are recruited during _____.
    In the presence of Ipi, _____ can be added at or slightly above the inflection point
    to prevent the alveoli from closing during expiration.

    A. inspiration; PEEP

    B. inspiration; tidal volume

    C. expiration; PEEP

    D. expiration; tidal volume

39. Over-inflation of the alveoli and _____ in C_{LT} leads to the appearance of an upper
    inflection point (Ipu). The Ipu can be minimized by reducing the _____.

    A. increase; PEEP

    B. increase; tidal volume

    C. decrease; PEEP

    D. decrease; tidal volume

40. On a flow-volume loop, the *expiratory* flow is _____ (above, below) the horizontal
    axis or volume measurement. The flow is usually _____ (increased, decreased)
    following bronchodilator therapy.

CHAPTER TWELVE

MANAGEMENT OF MECHANICAL VENTILATION

STRATEGIES TO IMPROVE VENTILATION

1. Alveolar hypoventilation causes respiratory _____ (acidosis, alkalosis) and it leads to _____ (bradycardia, hypoxemia, metabolic alkalosis) if supplemental oxygen is not provided to the patient.

2. A 45-year-old postoperative patient has the following blood gases: pH = 7.32, $PaCO_2$ = 55 mm Hg, PaO_2 = 58 mm Hg. The ventilatory status of this patient can be interpreted as _____ (hyperventilation, hypoventilation).

3. For COPD patients, the acceptable $PaCO_2$ range is from _____ (30 to 40, 40 to 50, 50 to 60) mm Hg due to _____ (acute, chronic) carbon dioxide retention.

4. Another method to assess the acceptable $PaCO_2$ in COPD patients is to review the patient's $PaCO_2$ obtained at the time of the _____ (current admission to, most recent discharge from) the hospital.

5. A patient who is on the ventilator during postoperative recovery has a recent $PaCO_2$ of 54 mm Hg. The physician wants to reduce the $PaCO_2$ to near 40 mm Hg. The most common method to achieve this is to:

   A. increase the mechanical rate.

   B. decrease the mechanical tidal volume.

   C. decrease the pressure support level.

   D. increase the mechanical deadspace.

6. When the mechanical rate is over 20/min, the incidence of _____ (pneumothorax, air leak, atelectasis, auto-PEEP) is increased, especially when pressure support ventilation is also used.

7. Minute Ventilation = (Ventilator V_T × Ventilator RR) + (Spontaneous V_T × Spontaneous RR). Based on the equation above, the minute ventilation can be increased by all of the following strategies *except*:

   A. increase the ventilator V_T.

   B. increase the ventilator RR.

   C. increase the spontaneous V_T.

   D. decrease the spontaneous RR.

8. Why is it undesirable to increase the ventilator tidal volume to increase the minute ventilation or to reduce the $PaCO_2$?

_____

_____

_____

9. A patient who is on the ventilator at a SIMV rate of 10/min has a $PaCO_2$ of 52 mm Hg. The physician wants to reduce the $PaCO_2$ to 40 mm Hg. Using the equation below, what is the estimated new SIMV rate to achieve this desired $PaCO_2$? [Assume the patient's spontaneous rate and tidal volume are stable.]

New rate = (Rate $\times$ $PaCO_2$) / Desired $PaCO_2$

A. 9/min

B. 11/min

C. 13/min

D. 15/min

10. The patient can help to improve the minute ventilation by _____ (increasing, decreasing) the spontaneous _____ (V_T only, RR only, V_T or RR).

11. During respiratory stress or when the ventilatory demand is high, a patient usually tries to increase the minute ventilation by _____ (increasing, decreasing) the spontaneous tidal volume.

12. A breathing pattern consisting of $\uparrow V_T$ and $\downarrow RR$ is _____ (more, less) advantageous than one of $\downarrow V_T$ and $\uparrow RR$ because a breathing pattern consisting of low tidal volume and high respiratory rate _____ (increases, decreases) the dead space ventilation.

13. During weaning attempts, for patients who are unable to maintain prolonged spontaneous ventilation or to overcome airway resistance, _____ (PEEP, 100% oxygen, pressure support ventilation) should be tried.

14. The level of pressure support is usually started at _____ (10 to 15, 15 to 20, 20 to 25) cm H_2O and it is adjusted until the spontaneous tidal volume _____ (increases, decreases) to an acceptable level.

15. Some practitioners prefer to titrate the pressure support level until the spontaneous respiratory rate is _____ (increased, reduced) to a desirable level. This change is usually observed in conjunction with a(n) _____ (increase, decrease) of the spontaneous tidal volume.

16. When pressure support ventilation is used properly, it reduces the work of breathing by increasing the spontaneous _____ (tidal volume, respiratory rate). As a result of this change, the spontaneous respiratory rate is often _____ (increased, decreased).

17. Pressure support ventilation increases spontaneous tidal volume, and therefore the minute ventilation.

(TRUE/FALSE)

18. The ventilator tidal volume is usually set according to the patient's _____ (body surface area, body weight) and the range available for adjustments is _____ (very broad, rather narrow).

19. Describe the potential effect of using (A) an excessive ventilator tidal volume, (B) insufficient ventilator tidal volume.

    (A) _____

    (B) _____

20. The minute ventilation may also be increased by using ventilator circuits with _____ (high, low) compressible volume.

21. High frequency jet ventilation has been used successfully to improve ventilation in _____ (infants, adults).

22. Why are patients with extremely high airway resistance or low compliance more likely to develop ventilator-related lung injuries?

    _____

    _____

23. Permissive hypercapnia is a strategy used to minimize the occurrence of ventilator-related lung injuries caused by positive pressure ventilation. It is done by selecting a tidal volume within the range of _____ to _____ ml/kg compared to the normal range of _____ to _____ ml/kg. The _____ (pH, $PaCO_2$, PaO_2) levels are allowed to increase beyond normal limits when this strategy is used.

24. The incidence of ventilator-induced lung injuries may be reduced by keeping the _____ (peak airway pressure, plateau pressure, PEEP) below 35 cm H_2O.

25. The small tidal volume used in permissive hypercapnia often causes alveolar _____ (hyperventilation, hypoventilation), CO_2 retention, and _____ (acidosis, alkalosis).

26. Severe acidosis may cause all of the following conditions *except*:
    A. decreased pulmonary vascular resistance.
    B. central nervous dysfunction.
    C. intracranial hypertension.
    D. neuromuscular weakness.

27. The acidosis associated with permissive hypercapnia may be corrected by all of the following *except*:
    A. renal compensation.
    B. administration of bicarbonate.
    C. administration of tromethamine.
    D. administration of glucocorticoid.

STRATEGIES TO IMPROVE OXYGENATION

28. A recent arterial blood gas report of a bronchitic patient shows mild hypoxemia. The initial method to improve the patient's oxygenation status is to:
    A. increase the F_IO_2.
    B. improve the cardiac output.
    C. start CPAP.
    D. use high frequency ventilation.

29. Oxygen therapy corrects uncomplicated hypoxemia because a higher F_IO_2 _____ (increases, decreases) the alveolar-capillary oxygen pressure gradient and enhances the diffusion of _____ (oxygen, carbon dioxide) from the lungs into the pulmonary circulation.

30. Oxygen therapy is very effective in correcting hypoxemia due to _____ (simple V/Q mismatch, intrapulmonary shunting, cardiac arrest).

31. Given: a/A ratio = 0.45. If a PaO_2 of 80 mm Hg is desired, what should be the PAO_2 and F_IO_2 needed? Use Equation 1 below to calculate the PAO_2 needed and Equation 2 for the F_IO_2 needed.

    Equation 1: PAO_2 needed = PaO_2 desired / (a/A ratio)

    Equation 2: F_IO_2 = [(PAO_2 needed) + 50] / 713

    A. PAO_2 = 118; F_IO_2 = 24%
    B. PAO_2 = 178; F_IO_2 = 32%
    C. PAO_2 = 216; F_IO_2 = 37%
    D. PAO_2 = 322; F_IO_2 = 52%

32. Hypoxemia that is due to hypoventilation may be corrected by oxygen therapy.

    (TRUE/ FALSE)

33. Hypoventilation is evident when the _____ (pH, $PaCO_2$, PaO_2) is _____ (less than 7.25, greater than 50 mm Hg, less than 50 mm Hg).

34. A 30-year-old patient who is breathing spontaneously at a rate of 28/min has blood gases as follows: pH = 7.22, $PaCO_2$ = 58 mm Hg, PaO_2 = 45 mm Hg. The physician wants to improve the patient's blood gases. Which of the following methods is most beneficial for this patient?
    A. oxygen therapy
    B. ventilation
    C. bicarbonate
    D. oxygen therapy and ventilation

35. Mild hypoxemia that is caused by _____ (shunting, dead space ventilation, hypoventilation) may be treated by improving the ventilation.

36. Refractory hypoxemia is usually caused by _____ (dead space ventilation, intrapulmonary shunting) and it _____ (does, does not) respond very well to oxygen therapy alone.

37. The treatment for refractory hypoxemia consists of a combination of all of the following *except*:
    A. oxygen.
    B. hyperbaric oxygen therapy.
    C. continuous positive airway pressure (CPAP).
    D. positive end-expiratory pressure (PEEP).

38. Refractory hypoxemia responds _____ (poorly, well) to supplemental oxygen when used with CPAP or PEEP.

39. During oxygen therapy, excessive oxygen is to be avoided because of all of the following potential complications *except*:

    A. pulmonary hypertension.

    B. oxygen toxicity.

    C. ciliary impairment.

    D. lung damage.

40. Alveolar ventilation may be improved by _____ (increasing, decreasing) the V_T or respiratory rate or by _____ (increasing, decreasing) the dead space ventilation.

41. In _____ (absolute, relative) hypovolemia, the problem is primarily due to volume loss and the treatment consists of fluid replacement.

42. In _____ (absolute, relative) hypovolemia, the problem is primarily due to loss of venous tone. Fluid replacement should be done with extreme caution because of the potential of fluid _____ (overload, depletion) when the vascular tone returns to normal.

43. Anemia may lead to hypoxia because majority (98%) of the oxygen in blood is carried by the _____ (plasma, platelets, hemoglobins).

44. Anemic hypoxia is likely when the hemoglobin level is less than _____ gm/100 ml of blood.

45. Continuous Positive Airway Pressure (CPAP) is useful in the treatment of refractory hypoxemia due to _____.

46. CPAP is only suitable for patients who have adequate _____ (heart, lung) mechanics and can sustain prolonged _____ (cardiac stress, spontaneous breathing).

47. Positive End-Expiratory Pressure (PEEP) is similar to CPAP with the exception that PEEP is used in conjunction with _____ (spontaneous breathing, mechanical ventilation).

48. CPAP and PEEP improve oxygenation by increasing a patient's _____ (tidal volume, vital capacity, functional residual capacity) and are therefore very useful in treating hypoxemia due to _____ (dead space ventilation, intrapulmonary shunting).

49. The table below shows the results obtained from the titration of optimal PEEP using pulse oximetry oxygen saturation (SpO_2) as the indicator. Based on these data, the optimal PEEP is _____ (0, 4, 7, 10, 12) cm H_2O. Explain why.

    _____

    _____

PEEP (cm H_2O)	SpO_2 (%)
0	81
4	85
7	91
10	89
12	87

50. During weaning of a patient who has been using 10 cm H_2O of PEEP and 70% oxygen, the _____ (PEEP, F_IO_2) should be reduced first until it reaches about _____ (5 cm H_2O, 40%). If the patient's vital signs remain stable, weaning of the other parameter may then begin.

51. A common application of inverse ratio ventilation (IRV) is for the treatment of patients with _____ (emphysema, asthma, ARDS) who are not responding to conventional _____ (oxygen therapy, CPAP, mechanical ventilation).

52. Inverse ratio ventilation improves oxygenation by overcoming the _____ (compliant, non-compliant) lung tissues, recruiting the _____ (over-distended, collapsed) alveoli, and _____ (increasing, decreasing) the time available for gas diffusion.

53. Extracorporeal membrane oxygenation (ECMO) is a method used to provide oxygenation of the blood _____ (within, outside) the body of an _____ (adult, infant).

ACID-BASE BALANCE

54. Mechanical ventilation may not be indicated in cases where a(n) _____ (increase, decrease) of $PaCO_2$ is a compensatory mechanism for metabolic _____ (acidosis, alkalosis).

55. Respiratory alkalosis is caused by alveolar _____ (hypoventilation, hyperventilation) and it may be the result of acute hypoxia or a compensatory mechanism for metabolic _____ (acidosis, alkalosis).

56. When respiratory alkalosis occurs during weaning from mechanical ventilation, the presence of hypoxia or metabolic acidosis must first be ruled out. Otherwise, reducing the rate on the ventilator will further induce _____ (hypoventilation, hyperventilation).

57. Ventilatory (respiratory) interventions _____ (should, should not) be used to compensate or correct primary metabolic problems.

TROUBLESHOOTING OF COMMON VENTILATOR ALARMS AND EVENTS

58. The low pressure alarms are triggered when the circuit pressure _____ (exceeds, drops below) the preset low pressure limit.

59. Factors that trigger the low pressure alarm usually _____ (will, will not) trigger the low volume alarm.

60. Conditions that may trigger the low pressure alarm include all of the following *except*:
    A. loss of circuit or system pressure.
    B. premature termination of inspiratory phase.
    C. obstruction of ventilator circuit.
    D. inappropriate ventilator settings.

61. The low expired volume alarm is triggered when the expired volume _____ (exceeds, drops below) the preset low volume limit.

62. The high pressure alarm is triggered when the ciruit pressure reaches or exceeds the preset _____ (high, low) pressure limit.

63. Conditions that may trigger the high pressure alarm include all of the following factors *except*:

    A. disconnection of ventilator circuit.

    B. increase of air flow resistance.

    C. decrease of lung compliance.

    D. decrease of chest wall compliance.

64. List at least three *mechanical* factors that may trigger the high pressure alarm due to an increase of air flow resistance.

    _____

    _____

65. List at least three *patient* factors that may trigger the high pressure alarm due to an increase of air flow resistance.

    _____

    _____

66. An acute and severe reduction of lung or chest wall compliance may also trigger the high pressure alarm. List at least three conditions that may cause a reduction of the lung or chest wall compliance.

    _____

    _____

67. The high respiratory rate alarm is triggered when the total rate _____ (exceeds, goes below) the high rate limit set on the ventilator. It may be triggered in all of the following conditions *except*:

    A. respiratory distress.

    B. excessive sensitivity setting.

    C. high rate alarm set too low.

    D. circuit disconnect.

68. In the event of frequent triggering of the high rate alarm, the high rate alarm may be set higher to disable the alarm.

    (TRUE/FALSE)

69. The apnea or low respiratory rate alarm is triggered when the total rate _____ (goes over, drops below) the low rate limit set on the ventilator.

70. All of the following conditions may trigger the apnea or low respiratory rate alarm *except*:

    A. respiratory distress.

    B. circuit disconnection.

    C. use of respiratory depressants.

    D. respiratory muscle fatigue.

71. The high PEEP alarm is triggered when the actual PEEP level _____ (exceeds, drops below) the preset PEEP limit.

72. Presence of excessive inadvertent PEEP may trigger the high PEEP alarm. All of the following conditions may lead to the development of inadvertent PEEP *except*:
    A. air trapping.
    B. inadequate inspiratory time.
    C. insufficient inspiratory flow.
    D. insufficient expiratory time.

73. Inadvertent PEEP caused by air trapping may be corrected by using a:
    A. higher ventilator rate.
    B. bronchodilator.
    C. lower inspiratory peak flow.
    D. longer inspiratory time.

74. The low PEEP alarm is triggered when the actual PEEP level _____ (goes over, drops below) the preset low PEEP limit. Failure of the ventilator circuit to hold the PEEP is usually due to _____ (obstruction, leakage) in the circuit or endotracheal tube cuff.

75. Auto-PEEP is commonly associated with _____ (CPAP, pressure support ventilation), significant air flow _____ (leakage, obstruction), respiratory rates of _____ (greater than, less than) 20/min, and _____ (excessive, insufficient) inspiratory flow rates.

CARE OF THE ARTIFICIAL AIRWAY

76. Patency of the ET tube can be maintained with adequate humidification and prompt removal of retained secretions.

    (TRUE/FALSE)

77. Since airway resistance is inversely related to the diameter of the tube, _____ (larger, smaller) endotracheal tubes cause an increased work of breathing.

78. According to Poiseuille's Law, when the radius of an airway is reduced by _____ (25%, 50%, 75%), the driving pressure (work of breathing) must be increased 16 times to maintain the same flow rate.

79. Proper function of the ciliary blanket of the airway is dependent on adequate _____ (oxygen, temperature, humidity).

80. Describe two methods to reduce the incidence of pulmonary contamination and infection during mechanical ventilation.

_____

_____

81 to 83. There are several potential sources of pathogens that can lead to pneumonia in the mechanically ventilated patient. Match the potential sources with the likely locations. Use each answer only once.

POTENTIAL SOURCE	LOCATIONS
81. Patient	A. Manual ventilation bag
82. Health care provider	B. Oropharynx
83. Equipment and supplies	C. Hands

84. The _____ (Gram stain, culture and sensitivity, acid-fast) method of sputum analysis is a technique used to quickly establish the general category of the suspected microbes so that appropriate broad-spectrum _____ may be administered.

85. Acid-fast sputum analysis is done to detect infection caused by _____ and silver stain is done to detect presence of _____ pneumonia.

86. _____ (Silver stain, Culture and sensitivity, Acid-fast) is done to identify the microbes in the sputum and select the most suitable antibiotics for the infection.

FLUID BALANCE

87. Fluid balance in the body is mainly affected by all of the following factors *except*:
    A. vascular and cellular fluid volume.
    B. pressure gradient of fluids.
    C. electrolyte balance.
    D. heart rate.

88. Water makes up about _____ (20, 40, 60, 80)% of the body weight with 20% of this volume distributed in the _____ (intracellular, extracellular) compartment and _____ % in the _____ (intracellular, extracellular) compartment.

89. When an excessive volume of fluid moves out of the extracellular compartment, an extracellular fluid _____ (surplus, deficit) occurs.

90. Mr. Williams, a patient admitted to the medical unit for tachycardia, hypotension, and decreased sensorium, is suspected to have extracellular fluid deficit. His problem may be caused by any of the following conditions *except*:
    A. dehydration.
    B. diarrhea.
    C. pulmonary edema.
    D. shifting of fluid into cells and tissues.

91. A(n) _____ (increase, decrease) of urine output is the most common sign of extracellular fluid deficit. This becomes evident when the urine output drops below _____ (20 ml/hr, 40 ml/hr, 60 ml/hr).

92. Oliguria or anuria is a _____ (central nervous, cardiovascular, renal) sign of extracellular fluid deficit.

93. The central nervous signs of extracellular fluid deficit include _____ and coma.

94. List at least three cardiovascular signs of extracellular fluid deficit.

_____

95. The treatment of extracellular fluid (ECF) deficit is _____ (potassium, plasma, fluid) replacement with Ringer's lactate solution since its composition is similar to the _____ (blood, ECF, urine).

96. A patient who has severe ECF deficit is being treated with fluid replacement therapy. What are the clinical signs that the treatment is successful?

_____

_____

97. Excessive fluid in the extracellular space is _____ (common, uncommon) in a clinical setting and it may lead to _____ (loss of sensorium, oliguria, pulmonary edema).

98. The treatment for excessive ECF is to _____ (administer, withhold) fluid or to give a(n) _____ (intravenous fluid, diuretic) such as furosemide.

99. _____ (Lasix, Mannitol) should not be used to treat ECF _____ (excess, deficit) because it can increase plasma volume before diuresis occurs.

100. Since use of diuretics to treat ECF excess will _____ (increase, decrease) the urine output, the volume of urine is therefore a _____ (good, poor) indicator of treatment success. Explain why.

_____

_____

101. A patient who has severe ECF excess is being treated with fluid restriction and diuretics. What are the clinical signs that the treatment is successful?

_____

_____

102. Diuresis often affects the electrolyte composition. For example, Lasix may lead to _____ (hyperkalemia, hypokalemia) and metabolic alkalosis whereas Diamox may _____ (increase, decrease) the serum bicarbonate level and cause _____ (acidosis, alkalosis).

ELECTROLYTE BALANCE

103. _____ is the major cation in the *extracellular* fluid compartment and it is directly related to the fluid level in the body. Its normal range is from _____ to _____ mEq/L.

104. _____ is the major cation in the *intracellular* fluid compartment and it is not related to the amount of fluid in the body. Its normal range is from _____ to _____ mEq/L.

105. The normal range for chloride ions in the plasma is from _____ to _____ mEq/L.

106. In most cases, once the sodium and potassium concentrations are properly managed and returned to normal, the chloride concentration will be corrected as well without further interventions.

    (TRUE/FALSE)

107. A patient has the following electrolyte values: Na^+ = 148 mEq/L, Cl^- = 99 mEq/L, HCO_3^- = 22 mEq/L. The anion gap is _____ mEq/L and it is _____ (normal, abnormal).

108. Muscle twitching, loss of reflexes, and increased intracranial pressure are three central nervous signs of _____ (hypernatremia, hyponatremia).

109. Restlessness, weakness, and delirium are three central nervous signs of _____ (hypernatremia, hyponatremia).

110. Fluids that contain no sodium _____ (should, should not) be used to correct fluid deficit. Explain why.

    _____

    _____

111. Hypernatremia is a(n) _____ (common, uncommon) problem and it is usually related to water _____ (excess, deficit) as a result of prolonged intravenous fluid administration with sufficient sodium but no dextrose.

112. The normal potassium concentration in plasma is from _____ to _____ mEq/L. It has a _____ (wide, narrow) normal range in the plasma because it is the major cation in the _____ (extracellular, intracellular) fluid.

113. Decreased muscle functions, flattened T wave and depressed ST segment on ECG, and decreased bowel activity are some clinical signs of _____ (hyperkalemia, hypokalemia).

114. Increased neuromuscular conduction, elevated T wave and depressed ST segment on ECG, and increased bowel activity are some clinical signs of _____ (hyperkalemia, hypokalemia).

115. Potassium deficiency may be caused by excessive K^+ loss as seen in all of the following conditions *except*:

    A. renal failure.

    B. trauma.

    C. severe infection.

    D. vomiting.

116. When potassium administration is needed, potassium chloride is commonly used because _____ (hyperchloremia, hypochloremia) usually co-exists with hypokalemia.

117. Potassium replacement via an intravenous route should be guided by all of the following conditions *except*:

    A. urine output should be at least 40 to 50 mL/hr.

    B. KCl should be undiluted.

    C. less than 200 mEq of potassium should be given in 24 hours.

    D. concentration of potassium should be less than 40 mEq/L.

118. What is the primary cause of hyperkalemia? Explain.

_____

_____

NUTRITION

119. Poor nutritional intake may indirectly result in all of the following *except*:
    A. depletion of muscle mass in diaphragm.
    B. respiratory muscle fatigue.
    C. hypocapnia.
    D. inability to wean.

120. Interstitial and pulmonary edema may develop in undernutritional status because severe hypoalbuminemia _____ (increases, decreases) the oncotic pressure and causes the fluid to shift into the _____ (cellular, interstitial) space.

121. Excessive nutrition or high caloric intake can cause respiratory distress due to _____ (increased, decreased) of oxygen consumption, and _____ (increased, decreased) carbon dioxide production.

122. A high-fat diet is more desirable than a high-carbohydrate diet for patients with CO_2 retention because the fat emulsion generates _____ (more, less) calories and _____ (more, less) carbon dioxide production.

123. Based on the Harris-Benedict equation for estimation of a patient's resting energy expenditure (REE) and total energy expenditure (TEE), _____ (more, less) calories are needed for patients under hypermetabolic or hypercatabolic conditions such as activity, trauma, infection, and burns.

124. Define hypophosphatemia.

_____

125. Describe the clinical signs of severe hypophosphatemia.

_____

_____

CHAPTER THIRTEEN

PHARMACOTHERAPY FOR MECHANICAL VENTILATION

DRUGS FOR IMPROVING VENTILATION

1. Airway narrowing is a common complication in patients receiving mechanical ventilation and it can cause varying degrees of respiratory distress. List at least three clinical signs of respiratory distress during mechanical ventilation.

   _____

   _____

2. During mechanical ventilation, some strategies that are useful in the management of airway narrowing include all of the following *except*:
   A. increasing the pressure limit.
   B. suctioning the endotracheal tube.
   C. administering bronchodilators.
   D. administering corticosteroids.

3. The sympathetic and parasympathetic nervous fibers are the basic subdivisions of the autonomic nervous system. Stimulation of the sympathetic branch results in _____ (bronchodilation, bronchoconstriction), whereas stimulation of the para-sympathetic branch causes _____ (bronchodilation, bronchoconstriction).

4. The neurotransmitter substance released at the *sympathetic* terminal axon is epinephrine (adrenaline) and it elicits a(n) _____ (adrenergic, cholinergic) response.

5. The neurotransmitter substance released at the terminal axon of the *parasympathetic* fiber is acetylcholine (ACh) and it elicits a(n) _____ (adrenergic, cholinergic) response.

6. Bronchodilation can be achieved by eliciting an adrenergic response. This is known as a _____ (sympathomimetic, parasympatholytic) action.

7. Bronchodilation can also be achieved by interfering with the cholinergic response. This is known as a _____ (sympathomimetic, parasympatholytic) action.

8. Adrenergic bronchodilators (Sympathomimetics) are agents that stimulate the adrenergic receptors via the sympathetic nerve fibers of the autonomic nervous system. The receptors thus stimulated include all of the following *except*:

   A. alpha 1 and alpha 2.

   B. beta 1.

   C. beta 2.

   D. omega 1.

9 to 12. Match the adrenergic receptors with the respective actions. Use each answer only once.

RECEPTOR	MAJOR EFFECTS
9. Alpha-1 (α-1) 10. Alpha-2 (α-2) 11. Beta-1 (β-1) 12. Beta-2 (β-2)	A. Positive **inotropic** effect ($\uparrow$ muscular contractility) Positive **chronotropic** effect ($\uparrow$ heart rate) B. Vasoconstriction Constriction of pupils C. Bronchodilation Peripheral vasodilation Decreased gastrointestinal activity D. Decreased gastrointestinal activity

13. Adrenergic bronchodilators are classified as catecholamines or catecholamine derivatives. Name at least two bronchodilators in each group.

   _____

   _____

14. Catecholamines have a _____ (rapid, slow) onset and undergo _____ (rapid, slow) degradation. They are _____ (effective, ineffective) when taken enterally.

15. Catecholamine derivatives are considered better bronchodilators than catecholamines. Describe the improved actions of these bronchodilators and explain what make the catecholamine derivatives better.

   _____

   _____

16. The adverse effects of adrenergic bronchodilators include all of the following *except*:

   A. tachycardia and palpitations.

   B. sleepiness.

   C. skeletal muscle tremors.

   D. nervousness.

17. Anticholinergic bronchodilators are agents that mainly _____ (enhance, impede) the impulses to the cholinergic receptors of the autonomic nervous system.

18. Atropine is a(n) _____ (cholinergic, anticholinergic) agent that is sometimes used as a secondary bronchodilator. Since it tends to _____ (increase, decrease) the heart rate, it is also used for symptomatic _____ (tachycardia, bradycardia).

19. The adverse effects of inhaled atropine aerosol include all of the following *except*:

    A. nervousness.

    B. headache.

    C. bradycardia.

    D. dried secretions.

20. Other anticholinergic agents such as ipratropium bromide (Atrovent) and glyco-pyrrolate (Robinul, an atropine derivative) are _____ (well, not well) absorbed systemically and when inhaled, produce _____ (more, fewer) adverse effects than those produced by atropine.

21. During acute episodes of bronchospasm where immediate response is required, ipratropium bromide is the preferred bronchodilator.

    (TRUE/FALSE)

22. Xanthine bronchodilators (theophylline and its salt form aminophylline) are use-ful in the management of airway narrowing associated with _____ (infection and trauma, asthma and COPD).

23. For individuals with carbon dioxide retention, xanthines _____ (improve, worsen) ventilation by _____ (heightening, diminishing) carbon dioxide sensi-tivity in the central nervous system and _____ (improving, hindering) diaphrag-matic contractility.

24. The three proposed mechanisms of action of theophylline are: _____ (produc-tion, inhibition) of phosphodiesterase, acting as an adenosine _____ (agonist, antagonist), and _____ (increased, decreased) catecholamine release.

25. Xanthines are commonly given via the inhalation route due to their ability to pen-etrate the mucosal lining of the airways.

    (TRUE/FALSE)

26. The initial signs of theophylline toxicity include all of the following *except*:

    A. nausea.

    B. vomiting.

    C. constipation.

    D. nervousness.

27. Theophylline toxicity may be avoided by keeping its serum level within _____ (1 to 10 μg/mL, 10 to 20 μg/mL, 20 to 30 μg/mL), the therapeutic range of theophylline.

28. Most of the theophylline is metabolized by the _____ (kidneys, liver, pancreas) and excreted in the urine. Patients at risk for theophylline toxicity are those with heart failure or _____ (renal, liver, pancreatic) disease.

29. Patients with diminished _____ (kidney, liver, pancreas) perfusion due to heart failure or impaired organ function can _____ (increase, reduce) the metabolism and clearance rate of theophylline. These patients are at risk of _____ (theo-phylline toxicity, bronchoconstriction) due to _____ (inadequate, excessive) serum theophylline level.

30. Patients who smoke _____ (increase, decrease) the level of hepatic enzyme and theophylline clearance. These patients therefore require a _____ (higher, lower) maintenance theophylline dosages to maintain bronchodilation.

31. Corticosteroids are potent _____ (bronchodilators, vitamins, blood components, hormones) that are released from the _____ (kidneys, liver, pancreas, adrenal cortex).

32. Corticosteroids are able to reduce _____ (agitation, inflammation, pulmonary edema) thus making them the drugs of choice in the management of chronic asthma and other similar airway conditions.

33. Corticosteroids have also been used successfully in all of the following conditions *except*:

    A. status asthmaticus.

    B. *Pneumocystis* pneumonia.

    C. drug-induced pneumonitis.

    D. ARDS.

34. Corticosteroids have _____ (strong, moderate, no) bronchodilator effect and _____ (should, should not) be given alone in status asthmaticus.

35. Corticosteroids have an onset time of about _____ (10 to 30 minutes, 1 to 2 hours, 2 to 24 hours).

36. Corticosteroids return constricted airways to normal by blocking the inflammatory mediators and they should be used when other traditional bronchodilators have failed to relieve bronchospasm.

    (TRUE/FALSE)

37. List the three general functions of corticosteroids.

    _____

38. In long-term use of aerosolized steroids, oral fungal infections (Candidiasis) often occur. They are usually caused by _____ and can be minimized by _____ the mouth after each aerosol treatment.

39. Systemic corticosteroids should be used cautiously with patients receiving steroidal based neuromuscular blocking agents (e.g., vecuronium bromide and pancuronium bromide) because of the potential of _____ (prolonged, shortened) blockade.

NEUROMUSCULAR BLOCKING AGENTS

40. Neuromuscular blocking agents are used to achieve all of the following goals *except*:

    A. calming the patient.

    B. relieving laryngeal spasm.

    C. providing muscle relaxation during surgery.

    D. easing management of airway and mechanical ventilation.

41. Other benefits of paralyzing agents include _____ (increased, reduced) chest wall compliance, _____ (increased, reduced) work of breathing, and _____ (increased, reduced) intracranial pressure.

42. Once a patient is paralyzed by a neuromuscular blocking agent, sedative drugs and narcotic analgesics are not necessary because the perception of pain does not exist with appropriate use of neuromuscular blocking drugs.

    (TRUE/FALSE)

43. At the neuromuscular junction, acetylcholine is the major chemical responsible for the transmission of nerve impulses. It is broken down by _____ stored in the vesicles.

44. When acetylcholine diffuses to the muscle end plate, it produces _____ (repolarization, depolarization) and muscle _____ (relaxation, contraction).

45. A repeating sequence of depolarization and repolarization is required for continued and coordinated muscular movement. Interruption at any point of the sequence causes muscle relaxation or paralysis, depending on the effective dosage.

    (TRUE/FALSE)

46. One type of neuromuscular blocker binds with the receptor site, producing quick onset and sustaining depolarization. This action _____ (facilitates, inhibits) subsequent neuromuscular transmission and renders further muscle contraction _____ (possible, impossible). Since these agents cause sustained depolarization, they are called _____ (depolarizing, nondepolarizing) agents.

47. There _____ (is no, are several) antidote(s) for depolarizing agents. The length of its neuromuscular blocking action is _____ (completely, partly) dependent on the degree of hydrolysis of succinylcholine by plasma pseudocholinesterase.

48. Another type of neuromuscular blocker competes with _____ for the receptor sites at the motor endplates, thus blocking the normal action of acetylcholine.

49. Since the nondepolarizing agents compete for the receptor sites, they are also called _____ agents.

50. Nondepolarizing blockers are antagonized by anticholinesterase and therefore the neuromuscular blocking action is _____ (reversible, irreversible).

51. _____ (Depolarizing, Nondepolarizing) agents have a quick onset but short duration of action, making them the drugs of choice for emergency intubation.

52. _____ (Depolarizing, Nondepolarizing) agents have longer onset times but they are also longer lasting. These drugs are more appropriate for neuromuscular blockade during controlled mechanical ventilation.

53. The degree of neuromuscular transmission and blockade of neuromuscular blocking agents may be influenced by all of the following factors except:
    A. organ failure.
    B. drug interaction.
    C. acid-base or electrolyte imbalance.
    D. Rh factor.

54. Patients with altered kidney and liver function have a(n) _____ (increased, decreased) risk of prolonged blockade because of _____ (increased, decreased) drug clearance and _____ (increased, decreased) drug accumulation.

55. Beta blockers, procainamide, quinidine, calcium channel blockers, and nitroglycerine may potentiate the effects of _____ (depolarizing, nondepolarizing) agents.

56. High concentrations of antibiotics may _____ (potentiate, diminish) the effects of competitive agents by decreasing the release of _____ (acetylcholine, anticholinesterase). A lower level of _____ (acetylcholine, anticholinesterase) makes the action of the competitive agents more _____ (intense, subdued).

57. Patients receiving systemic corticosteroids and steroidal based vecuronium bromide or pancuronium bromide may experience _____ (prolonged, shortened) blockade possibly related to the comparable chemical structure of these two agents.

58. Calcium functions to cause _____ (release, capture) of acetylcholine (ACh) from the vesicles. An increased level of calcium therefore _____ (enhances, diminishes) muscular contraction.

59. The action of magnesium works in opposition to calcium. An increased level of magnesium therefore _____ (increases, decreases) release of ACh and _____ (enhances, diminishes) muscular contraction.

60. Because of the respective action of calcium and magnesium on acetylcholine, low calcium and high magnesium levels can enhance the effects of _____ (depolarizing, nondepolarizing) agents. Low magnesium levels can magnify the effects of _____ (depolarizing, nondepolarizing) agents.

61. Hypokalemia causes a(n) _____ (increase, decrease) of neuromuscular blockade with nondepolarizing agents and a(n) _____ (increase, decrease) of neuromuscular blockade with depolarizing agents.

62. When neuromuscular blockers are used, acidemia _____ (intensifies, diminishes) neuromuscular blockade whereas alkalemia _____ (intensifies, diminishes) it.

63. Although many factors alter the action of neuromuscular blocking agents, proper individual dosage can be titrated after the initial dose by monitoring the patient and by meeting the clinical objectives set by the physician.

    (TRUE/FALSE)

64. The *most* serious adverse effect during use of neuromuscular blocking agents is:
    A. apnea.
    B. loss of coughing mechanism.
    C. muscle atrophy.
    D. psychological trauma.

65. Use of succinylcholine, tubocurarine, metocurine, and atracurium may provoke bronchospasm and hypotension due to release of _____ (acetylcholine, histamine, corticosteroid).

66. List at least three cardiovascular adverse effects of neuromuscular blocking agents.

    _____

    _____

67. The Train-of-Four is a peripheral nerve stimulator used to determine the degree of _____.

68. The ability to open eyes _____ (slightly, widely), sustain head _____ (nod, lift), and protrude the tongue for more than _____ (two, five) seconds are signs of adequate reversal of neuromuscular blockade.

69. Return of diaphragm function is accessed by acceptable blood gases, maximal inspiratory pressure (MIP) greater than _____ (–15, –25) cmH$_2$O, and vital capacity greater than _____ (300, 600, 900) mL.

SEDATIVES AND ANTI-ANXIETY AGENTS— BENZODIAZEPINES

70. Benzodiazepines are used in all of the following conditions *except* patients who are:
    A. having trouble breathing.
    B. very anxious about the intensive care environment.
    C. undergoing bronchoscopy procedure.
    D. very combative.

71. Gamma-aminobutyric acid (GABA) receptors are the major _____ (autonomic, central) nervous system inhibitory transmitters. Once the neurons are hyperpolarized by the GABA action, the neurons become _____ (more, less) resistant to repeated depolarization and sedation results.

72. Benzodiazepines _____ (facilitate, inhibit) the action of GABA thus producing clinical sedation, anxiolysis, anticonvulsant effects, amnesia, slower reaction time, visual accommodation difficulties, and ataxia.

73. Benzodiazepines are usually administered via the _____ (oral, intravenous, intramuscular) route because of unreliable _____ (gastrointestinal, venous) absorption. In addition, pain and _____ (fast, slow) onset of action are associated with _____ (oral, intravenous, intramuscular) administration.

74. Benzodiazepines are metabolized in the _____ (liver, kidneys, pancreas, gall bladder) into active and inactive metabolites which are excreted mainly in the urine.

75. In most clinical settings, the choice of benzodiazepine is often based on _____ (mode of action, speed of onset, duration of action, cost).

76. The physician is concerned about the adverse CNS effects of benzodiazepines on her patient and asks you to look for any signs of adverse effects. You would look for all of the following signs *except*:
    A. confusion.
    B. combativeness.
    C. drowsiness.
    D. syncope.

77. A patient who has been using benzodiazepines for several weeks is showing the following signs during the weaning attempt: anxiety, tachycardia, diaphoresis, hypertension, and some seizures. You would report to the physician that the patient might be experiencing:

    A. ventilatory failure.

    B. hypoxic brain syndrome.

    C. metabolic acidosis.

    D. withdrawal syndrome of benzodiazepines.

78. Parenteral administration of benzodiazepines may result in a dose-dependent respiratory _____ (stimulation, depression), especially when they are used in addition to _____ (corticosteroids, narcotics, bronchodilators).

79. As you are monitoring the hemodynamic status of a patient, you read in the chart that the patient has been given benzodiazepines for the management of mechanical ventilation. You would expect a(n):

    A. decrease of mean arterial pressure.

    B. increase of stroke volume.

    C. increase of cardiac output.

    D. increase of systemic vascular resistance.

80. Since individual response to benzodiazepines is highly _____ (predictable, variable), monitoring is _____ (not necessary, essential) to ensure correct dosing and low cost.

81. Using the Ramsay Scale for Assessment of Sedation, a patient who is cooperative and oriented would have a level/score of _____ (I, II, V, VI), whereas a patient who is asleep with sluggish response to stimulation would have a level/score of _____ (I, II, V, VI).

82. The Ramsay Scale is used to assess a patient's state of _____ (sedation, combativeness, airway reactivity) and it is not suitable for use in _____ (sedated, paralyzed) patients since they cannot perform those commands as required for the Ramsay Scale assessment.

83. To assess the degree of sedation in paralyzed patients, _____ (central nervous, autonomic nervous) signs such as tachycardia, diaphoresis, hypertension, and lacrimation may suggest _____ (excessive, inadequate) sedation or pain control.

84 to 86. Match each benzodiazepine with its respective onset and duration of action. Use each answer only once.

DRUG	ONSET/DURATION
84. Diazepam (Valium) 85. Lorazepam (Ativan) 86. Midazolam (Versed)	A. Fast onset / Duration is short but may be prolonged if not carefully dosed. B. Fast onset / Duration is short initially; multiple doses result in prolonged effect. C. Intermediate onset / Duration is intermediate.

NARCOTIC ANALGESICS

87 to 91. Severe pain may lead to many different physiological reactions. Match the reactions with the respective adverse outcomes. Use each answer only once.

REACTION INDUCED BY PAIN	SELECTED ADVERSE OUTCOMES
87. Tissue initiated stress hormone response	A. Delay of bowel and gastric function
88. Activation of autonomic functions	
89. Muscle splinting	B. Formation of deep vein thrombosis and pulmonary embolism
90. Immobility	
91. Diminished gastrointestinal function	C. Increase of blood pressure and heart rate
	D. Breakdown of body tissue and increase of blood clotting
	E. Decrease of ventilatory efficiency and hypoventilation

92. Narcotic analgesics produce analgesia by binding to opioid receptors (e.g., mu, kappa, and sigma receptors) in and outside the _____ (autonomic nervous, central nervous) system.

93. Describe the primary CNS effects caused by activiation of the mu, kappa, and sigma receptors.

_____

_____

94. Opiates may be further classified depending on whether they are agonists, agonist-antagonists, or antagonists. Opiates that produce a maximal response within cells to which they bind are called _____ (agonists, agonist-antagonists, antagonists) and those that only block opiate receptors are known as _____ (agonists, agonist-antagonists, antagonists).

95. Morphine, meperidine, and fentanyl are examples of _____ (agonists, agonist-antagonists, antagonists).

96. Naloxone (Narcan) is an example of an _____ (agonist, agonist-antagonist, antagonist).

97. Antagonist drugs such as naloxone (Narcan) are primarily used to _____ (intensify, reverse) the effects of narcotics. When they are used on patients being treated with narcotics, they may _____ (cause, reverse) respiratory depression and lead to the return of _____ (severe pain, spontaneous breathing, severe pain and spontaneous breathing).

98. List the adverse effects of narcotic analgesics on the central nervous system.

_____

_____

99. Myoclonus (twitching or spasm of muscles), convulsions, and chest wall rigidity are the primary adverse effects of narcotic analgesics on the muscle group.

(TRUE/FALSE)

100. The cardiovascular effects of narcotic analgesics include all of the following *except*:
    A. direct vasoconstriction.
    B. histamine release.
    C. bradycardia.
    D. hypotension.

101. One method to prevent hypotension induced by narcotic analgesics is to:
    A. use the highest effective dose.
    B. provide a diuretic.
    C. increase the rate of drug administration.
    D. combine low dose narcotic and sedative.

102. Fast gastric emptying, diarrhea, and vomiting are the primary adverse effects of narcotic analgesics on the GI system.

    (TRUE/FALSE)

103. Other effects related to opioid use include _____ (dilation, contraction) of pupils, altered levels of stress hormones, and uncommon allergic reactions.

104. The precipitation of a withdrawl syndrome upon abrupt termination of a drug or after administration of a narcotic antagonist is called _____ (tolerance, physical dependence, psychological dependence).

105. A physician is concerned about the level of pain that his patient may have during mechanical ventilation. He asks you to look for signs of pain. You would look for all of the following clinical signs *except*:
    A. bradycardia.
    B. blood pressure changes.
    C. diaphoresis.
    D. guarding.

AGENTS FOR SEIZURES AND ELEVATED INTRACRANIAL PRESSURE (BARBITURATES)

106. Explain why barbiturates have limited applications in patients on mechanical ventilation.

    _____

    _____

107. Barbiturates may be preferred in all of the following situations *except*:
    A. seizure disorders.
    B. control of elevated intracranial pressure.
    C. management of pain.
    D. rapid sequence intubation.

108. Since an effective hypnotic dose of phenobarbital lasts _____ (1 to 4, 2 to 8, 4 to 12) hours, it is considered a _____ (short-acting, intermediate-acting, long-acting) drug.

109. Barbiturates depress the CNS function via the GABA mediated hyperpolarization of the neuron, making the neuron _____ (more, less) resistant to depolarization.

110. Barbiturates cause _____ (venoconstriction, venodilation) with peripheral pooling of blood, tachycardia, and depressed myocardial contractility. These events may result in _____ (hypertension, hypotension) especially in elderly patients with _____ (adequate, inadequate) cardiac function.

111. List at least three adverse respiratory effects caused by use of barbiturates.

_____

_____

112. Barbiturates _____ (increase, decrease) the clearance of drugs that are metabolized by the liver, thus _____ (increasing, decreasing) the effects of those drugs.

113. Barbiturates _____ (do, do not) relieve pain and may sometimes _____ (heighten, depress) the sensation of pain.

OTHER AGENTS USED IN MECHANICAL VENTILATION

114. Other agents commonly used in mechanical ventilation include propofol (for sedation and maintenance of _____), haloperidol (for sedation and reduction of _____), and nitric oxide (for dilation of _____).

115. Propofol (Diprivan) is an _____ (oral, intravenous, intramuscular) drug administered together with other anesthetics to produce and maintain anesthesia.

116. The mode of action of propofol is believed to be the _____ (enhancement, reduction) of GABA-activated chloride ion channel function.

117. Adverse reactions of propofol include all of the following *except*:
    A. apnea.
    B. tachycardia.
    C. airway constriction.
    D. hypotension.

118. How does propofol contribute to a patient's total caloric intake?

_____

_____

119. Since fat emulsion provides an excellent medium for microbial growth, strict aseptic techniques are essential when propofol is used.

    (TRUE/FALSE)

120. Propofol has _____ (no, moderate, potent) analgesic properties and additional analgesics are _____ (often, sometimes, seldomly) needed for adequate pain control.

121. Propofol _____ (does, does not) promote salivation or vomiting. Its use can be a(n) _____ (advantage, disadvantage) for intubated patients.

122. The infusion rate of propofol should be reduced _____ (rapidly, gradually) to reduce the effects of pain and disorientation.

123. Before haloperidol (Haldol) is used on a ventilator patient presenting with delirium, a search for the reversible causes of delirium should first be done. Explain why.

_____

_____

124. Once other causes are ruled out, haloperidol is used for the control of _____.

125. Haloperidol (Haldol) may be given by:
    A. intravenous route.
    B. intramuscular route.
    C. oral route.
    D. all of the above.

126. Agitation and delirium are likely caused by a(n) _____ (increase, decrease) in dopamine release and metabolism. Haloperidol produces a calming effect by _____ (blocking, facilitating) the dopamine receptors in the central nervous system.

127. What is the primary adverse effect of blockade of dopamine receptors?

_____

128. Haloperidol may also prolong the electrocardiographic _____ (ST, QT, QRS) interval that on rare occasions can produce torsade de pointes, a polymorphic form of ventricular _____ (fibrillation, tachycardia).

129. Combined use of benzodiazepine, opioid, and haloperidol is often necessary for control of extremely agitated, delirious patients.

    (TRUE/FALSE)

130. Inhaled nitric oxide (NO) therapy is currently being evaluated for its potential application in all of the following conditions *except*:
    A. congenital heart disease.
    B. persistent pulmonary hypertension of the newborn.
    C. pleural effusion.
    D. respiratory distress syndrome.

131. Inhaled nitric oxide produces local _____ (vasodilation, vasoconstriction) of vascular smooth muscles in the lung and it reduces pulmonary vascular resistance, corrects V/Q mismatch, and improves oxygenation.

132. Why are the by-products of nitric oxide harmful to the lungs?

_____

_____

133. Nitric oxide is inactivated by combining with hemoglobin to form _____, a form of hemoglobin in blood that is incapable of transporting oxygen.

CHAPTER FOURTEEN

WEANING FROM MECHANICAL VENTILATION

DEFINITION OF WEANING SUCCESS AND FAILURE

1. Weaning success is defined as effective spontaneous breathing _____ (with some, without any) mechanical assistance for _____ (2, 12, 24) hours or more.

2. The time needed to wean medical patients is generally _____ (longer, shorter) than surgical patients since medical patients often have _____ (more, less) co-existing complicating problems.

3. Patients who fail the weaning process usually have abnormal blood gases at the _____ (beginning, end) of the weaning trial or clinical deterioration to an unacceptable state. List at least three signs that indicate deterioration of clinical condition.

   _____

4. Weaning failure may be defined as return of the patient to mechanical ventilation after _____ (2 hours, 12 hours, any length) of weaning trial.

PATIENT CONDITION PRIOR TO WEANING

5. Before a weaning trial is begun, the patient should be _____ (partially, fully) recovered from the condition resulting in ventilatory support and be able to assume _____ (oxygenation, spontaneous breathing).

6 to 8. Match the conditions that may hinder weaning success with the respective examples. Use each answer only once.

CONDITIONS	EXAMPLES
6. Patient/Pathophysiologic	A. pH imbalance, severe anion gap
7. Cardiac/Circulatory	B. Fever, infection, sleep deprivation
8. Dietary/Acid-base/Electrolytes	C. Arrhythmias, abnormal blood pressures, hypotension

WEANING CRITERIA

9. Weaning criteria are used to evaluate the:
   A. readiness of a patient to begin the weaning trial.
   B. likelihood of weaning success.
   C. readiness for extubation.
   D. A and B only.

10. Weaning is more likely to succeed if a patient meets _____ (one or two, most) of the weaning criteria.

11 to 15. Write in the normal values or normal ranges for each of the following *ventilatory* weaning criteria.

VENTILATORY WEANING CRITERIA	NORMAL VALUES/RANGES
11. $PaCO_2$	< _____ mm Hg with normal pH
12. Vital capacity	> _____ to _____ ml/kg
13. Spontaneous V_T	> _____ to _____ ml/kg
14. Spontaneous RR (f)	< _____ /min
15. Spontaneous resting minute ventilation	< _____ L

16 to 21. Write in the normal values for each of the following *oxygenation* weaning criteria.

OXYGENATION WEANING CRITERIA	NORMAL VALUES
16. PaO_2 (without PEEP)	> _____ mm Hg @ F_IO_2 up to 0.4
17. PaO_2 (with PEEP)	> _____ mm Hg @ F_IO_2 up to 0.4
18. SaO_2	> _____ @ F_IO_2 up to 0.4
19. Q_S/Q_T	< _____ %
20. $P(A-a)O_2$	< _____ mm Hg @ F_IO_2 of 1.0
21. PaO_2/F_IO_2	> _____ mm Hg

22 to 23. Write in the normal values for each of the following *pulmonary reserve* weaning criteria.

PULMONARY RESERVE WEANING CRITERIA	NORMAL VALUES / RANGES
22. Maximum Voluntary Ventilation	> _____ × min vent @ F_IO_2 up to 0.4
23. Maximum Inspiratory Pressure	> _____ to _____ cm H_2O in 20 sec

24 to 25. Write in the normal values for each of the following *pulmonary measurement* weaning criteria.

PULMONARY MEASUREMENT WEANING CRITERIA	NORMAL VALUES
24. Static Compliance	> _____ ml/cm H_2O
25. V_D/V_T	< _____ %

26. The partial pressure of carbon dioxide in the arterial blood ($PaCO_2$) is the most reliable indicator of a patient's _____ (oxygenation, acid-base, ventilatory) status.

27. Weaning from mechanical ventilation should be attempted only when the $PaCO_2$ is between _____ and _____ mm Hg with a _____ (acidotic, compensated, alkalotic) pH. The $PaCO_2$ may be _____ (higher, lower) for COPD patients.

28. Explain why it is desirable to allow the patient to breath spontaneously for one to two minutes prior to measuring the vital capacity and spontaneous tidal volume.

   _____

   _____

29. The _____ (tidal volume, vital capacity) measurement is effort dependent. Valid measurements of this weaning parameter _____ (require, do not require) proper explanation and coaching.

30. For a successful weaning outcome, the spontaneous respiratory rate should be _____ (more than, less than) 30 to 35 breaths per minute while the corresponding $PaCO_2$ should be _____ (more than, less than) 50 mm Hg.

31. A _____ (rapid, slow) breathing pattern is a sign of respiratory distress and it reflects _____ (good, poor) readiness for weaning trial.

32. The patient's spontaneous resting minute volume should be _____ (more, less) than 10 liters per minute for a successful weaning outcome because a _____ (high, low) minute ventilation requirement implies that the work of breathing is _____ (excessive, minimal).

33. An excessive minute volume requirement may be caused by a(n) _____ (increased, decreased) carbon dioxide production secondary to metabolic _____ (acidosis, alkalosis), or a(n) _____ (increased, decreased) metabolic rate or alveolar dead space.

34. Causes of a(n) _____ (increased, decreased) carbon dioxide production include extensive burn injuries, an elevated body temperature and sometimes overfeeding, especially with _____ (fat, carbohydrate) dietary supplements.

35. PaO_2 and SaO_2 measurements _____ (do, do not) reflect the true oxygenation status of patients with anemia or increased levels of dysfunctional hemoglobins. Under these conditions, _____ (pulse oximetry saturation, arterial oxygen content, arterial pH) should be measured and used to evaluate the oxygenation status.

36. The physiologic shunt to total perfusion (Q_S/Q_T) ratio is used to estimate how much _____ (ventilation, pulmonary perfusion) is wasted. An increased Q_S/Q_T ratio usually leads to _____ (hypercapnia, hypoxemia, acidosis).

37. A patient has the following oxygen content measurements: CcO_2 = 20 vol%, CaO_2 = 18 vol%, CvO_2 = 13 vol%. The calculated Q_S/Q_T is about _____ and it reflects _____ shunting.

   A. 10%, mild

   B. 29%, significant

   C. 35%, severe

   D. 65%, severe

38. A patient is being assessed for weaning trial and the blood gas parameters are as follows: $F_IO_2 = 100\%$, $PAO_2 = 654$ mm Hg, $PaO_2 = 197$ mm Hg. The calculated $P(A-a)O_2$ is _____ and the estimated shunt is _____.
    A. 457 mm Hg, 23%
    B. 457 mm Hg, 45%
    C. 851 mm Hg, 23%
    D. 851 mm Hg, 45%

39. On a 100% inspired oxygen concentration, every 50 mm Hg difference in $P(A-a)O_2$ approximates _____ (1, 2, 5)% physiologic shunt.

40. The arterial oxygen tension to inspired oxygen concentration (PaO_2/F_IO_2) index is a simplified method for estimating the degree of _____ (dead space ventilation, ventilation/perfusion mismatch, intrapulmonary shunt).

41. A PaO_2/F_IO_2 index of 200 mm Hg or _____ (higher, lower) is indicative of normal physiologic shunt and compatible to successful weaning trial.

42. Vital capacity (VC) and maximum inspiratory pressure (MIP) are two weaning criteria that are used to reflect a patient's _____ ($PaCO_2$, PaO_2, pulmonary reserve).

43. Explain why proper explanation and coaching is important before obtaining the VC and MIP measurements.

    _____

    _____

44. Vital capacity measures the maximum amount of lung volume that the patient can exhale following _____ (tidal inspiration, maximal inspiration).

45. For a more successful weaning outcome, the patient should have a VC of greater than _____ to _____ ml/kg.

46. Maximum inspiratory pressure is the amount of _____ (positive, negative) pressure that a patient can generate in 20 seconds when inspiring against an _____ (opened, occluded) pressure manometer.

47. For a more successful weaning outcome, the patient should be able to generate an MIP of greater than _____ cm H_2O.

48. A patient's work of breathing is increased in conditions of _____ (high, low) compliance, _____ (high, low) airway resistance, and _____ (high, low) V_D/V_T ratio.

49. The static lung compliance is calculated by dividing the patient's tidal volume by the difference in the _____ (peak airway, plateau) pressure and the PEEP.

50. A static compliance value of 30 ml/cm H_2O or _____ (greater, less) is consistent with a readiness to begin the weaning process.

51. The airway resistance is calculated by dividing the difference in the _____ (peak airway, plateau) pressure and the (plateau pressure, PEEP) by the constant inspiratory flow.

52. _____ (PEEP, Pressure controlled ventilation, Pressure support ventilation) is effective in reducing the circuit and airway resistance during spontaneous breathing.

53. The V_D/V_T ratio estimates the volume of each breath that is being perfused by pulmonary circulation.

    (TRUE/ FALSE)

54. The blood gases and related parameters of a patient are as follows: pH = 7.43, $PaCO_2$ = 40 mm Hg, PaO_2 = 80 mm Hg, $PECO_2$ = 30 mm Hg. What portion of the tidal volume is considered wasted?

    A. 25%

    B. 50%

    C. 75%

    D. none of the above

COMBINED WEANING INDEX

55. Unlike weaning criteria that are typically used to assess a patient's _____ (readiness to wean, weaning success), combined weaning indices are used to predict _____ (readiness to wean, weaning success).

56 to 58. In the table below, write in the normal threshold for each of the combined weaning indices.

COMBINED WEANING INDEX	NORMAL THRESHOLD FOR SUCCESSFUL WEANING
56. Respiratory Frequency to Tidal Volume Ratio (f/V_T) (Rapid Shallow Breathing Index)	< _____ breaths/min/L
57. Simplified Weaning Index (SWI)	< _____ /min
58. Compliance Rate Oxygenation and Pressure (CROP) Index	> _____ ml/cycles/min

59. Shallow breathing leads to _____ (efficient, inefficient) ventilation because the anatomic dead space volume contributes to a _____ (larger, lower) V_D/V_T ratio when the tidal volume is reduced.

60. A large f/V_T ratio indicates _____ (efficient, inefficient) ventilation. Therefore a successful weaning outcome should have a f/V_T ratio of _____ (more than, less than) < 100 cycles/L.

61. Describe the procedure to measure the f/V_T ratio.

    _____

    _____

    _____

    _____

62. A patient who is being considered for weaning has these measurements obtained during spontaneous breathing: V_E = 4.2 L/min, f = 16/min. What is the patient's f/V_T ratio? Does the ratio predict a successful weaning outcome?

    A. 38; successful weaning outcome

    B. 61; successful weaning outcome

    C. 38; unsuccessful weaning outcome

    D. 61; unsuccessful weaning outcome

63. Calculation of the simplified weaning index requires all of the following information *except*:

    A. ventilator respiratory rate (fmv).

    B. ventilator pressure readings.

    C. maximum inspiratory pressure (MIP).

    D. $PaCO_2$ during spontaneous breathing.

64. When the calculated simplified weaning index (SWI) is less than _____ /min, it is highly predictive of weaning success.

65. When the calculated simplified weaning index (SWI) is more than _____ /min, it is highly predictive of weaning failure.

66. A patient has the following measurements before a weaning attempt. What is the calculated simplified weaning index (SWI)? Does it predict a successful weaning outcome?

    f_{mv}: 6/min, PIP = 45 cm H_2O, PEEP = 5 cm H_2O, MIP = –30 cm H_2O, $PaCO_2$ mv = 40 mm Hg.

    A. SWI = 8/min, predictive of weaning success

    B. SWI = 10/min, predictive of weaning success

    C. SWI = 8/min, predictive of weaning failure

    D. SWI = 10/min, predictive of weaning failure

67. The Compliance Rate Oxygenation and Pressure (CROP) weaning index includes all of the following measurements *except*:

    A. static compliance (CST).

    B. spontaneous respiratory rate (f).

    C. arterial PO_2 to alveolar PO_2 (PaO_2/PAO_2) ratio.

    D. maximum inspiratory pressure (MIP).

68. CROP index evaluates a patient's pulmonary gas exchange and the balance between respiratory demands and respiratory neuromuscular reserve. Pulmonary gas exchange is reflected by the _____ (C_{DYN}, MIP, PaO_2/PAO_2, f). Respiratory demand is shown by the _____ (C_{DYN}, MIP, PaO_2/PAO_2, f). The respiratory and muscular reserve is shown by the C_{DYN} and _____ (MIP, PaO_2/PAO_2, f).

69. A CROP index of _____ ml/breaths/min or _____ (higher, lower) is predictive of weaning success.

70. A patient who has been on the ventilator for about three weeks is being evaluated for a weaning attempt. The latest CROP measurements are as follows: C_{DYN} = 25 ml/cm H_2O, MIP = –20 cm H_2O, PaO_2/PAO_2 = 0.6, f = 20 breaths/min. What is the CROP index? Does it predict weaning success?

    A. 12 ml/breaths/min, predictive of weaning success

    B. 15 ml/breaths/min, predictive of weaning success

    C. 12 ml/breaths/min, predictive of weaning failure

    D. 15 ml/breaths/min, predictive of weaning failure

WEANING PROCEDURE

71. Weaning with aerosol T-tube is done by alternating T-tube and mechanical ventilation with progressively more time on _____ (the T-tube, mechanical ventilation) and less time on _____ (the T-tube, mechanical ventilation).

72. Weaning with SIMV is done by progressively _____ (increasing, decreasing) the *mandatory* rate of the _____ (patient, ventilator), usually _____ to _____ breaths per min at each step.

73. The pace of mandatory rate reduction during SIMV weaning is dictated by the _____ (insurance policy, RT department policy, patient's tolerance).

74. Pressure support ventilation (PSV) is useful during weaning attempts because it reduces the _____ (compliance, airway resistance) imposed on the patient by the endotracheal tube and ventilator circuit.

75. Weaning with pressure support ventilation is done by starting the pressure support level at _____ to _____ cm H_2O and adjusting it gradually up to a maximum of _____ cm H_2O.

76. The pressure support level is titrated until a desired _____ or _____ is obtained.

SIGNS OF WEANING FAILURE

77. The weaning process should be _____ (continued, stopped) if the patient shows signs of muscle fatigue or ventilatory failure.

78. As you are monitoring a patient who is being weaned off the ventilator, you notice that the patient exhibits some unusual clinical signs during prolonged spontaneous breathing. You would notify the physician of the following early signs of weaning failure *except*:
    A. eucapnic ventilation.
    B. use of accessory muscles.
    C. paradoxical abdominal movements.
    D. diaphoresis.

79 to 81. Complete the following indicators of weaning failure.

INDICATORS	EXAMPLES
79. Blood Gases	Increasing $PaCO_2$ to > _____ mm Hg Decreasing pH to < _____ Decreasing PaO_2 to < _____ mm Hg Decreasing SpO_2 to < _____ %
80. Vital Signs	Changing blood pressures by _____ mm Hg systolic or _____ mm Hg diastolic Increasing heart rate by _____ /min, or > _____ /min
81. Respiratory Parameters	Decreasing V_T to < _____ ml Increasing RR (f) to > _____ /min Increasing RR/V_T (f/V_T) ratio to > _____ cycles/L Decreasing MIP to < _____ cm H_2O Decreasing static compliance to < _____ cm H_2O Increasing V_D/V_T to > _____ %

CAUSES OF WEANING FAILURE

82. List the three major causes of weaning failure.

   _____

   _____

83. To minimize the effect on air flow resistance, a size _____ or larger endotracheal tube should be used because its cross sectional area is similar to that of adult _____ (trachea, bronchus, glottis).

84. Another strategy to reduce the air flow resistance during mechanical ventilation is to cut the ET tube to about _____ (one centimeter, one inch, two inches) from the patient's lips or nares.

85. The section of ET tube that is cut should be _____ (discarded, displayed) prominently. Explain why.

   _____

   _____

86. Other causes of increased airway resistance during mechanical ventilation include all of the following conditions *except*:
   A. kinking of ET tube.
   B. secretions in ET tube.
   C. use of pulse oximeter.
   D. use of end-tidal CO_2 monitor probe.

87. The work of breathing may also be raised because of an increased _____ (oxygen, carbon dioxide) production secondary to a _____ (higher, lower) metabolic rate.

88. _____ (High, Low) lung or thoracic compliance makes lung expansion difficult and it is a major contributing factor to respiratory muscle fatigue and weaning failure.

89. List at least three clinical conditions that may lead to a decreased *static* compliance.

   _____

90. List at least three clinical conditions that may lead to a decreased *dynamic* compliance.

   _____

91. Work of Breathing = P_{TP} (transpulmonary pressure) × V_T (tidal volume)

   Based on the above equation, the work of breathing is increased when the transpulmonary pressure is _____ (increased, decreased).

92. The transpulmonary pressure is increased in conditions of _____ (high, low) compliance or _____ (high, low) airway resistance.

93. Persistent increase of the transpulmonary pressure may lead to respiratory muscle fatigue and eventual ventilatory failure.

   (TRUE/FALSE)

94. Respiratory muscle dysfunction may be due to all of the following conditions *except*:

    A. respiratory muscular atrophy due to muscle disuse.

    B. excessive nutritional intake.

    C. low oxygen delivery.

    D. electrolyte imbalance.

95. Describe two methods that may improve the functions of the respiratory muscles and diaphragms after prolonged mechanical ventilation and muscle disuse.

    _____

TERMINAL WEANING

96. Terminal weaning is defined as _____ (withholding, withdrawal) of mechanical ventilation which results in the death of a patient.

97. A patient's informed consent means that the patient agrees to have the life-sustaining devices removed and he/she understands the potential consequences, _____ (including, excluding) death.

98. Discussions on a patient's informed consent should be done _____ (during the physician rounds, over a period of time). Explain why.

    _____

    _____

99. Terminal weaning may be justified if medical intervention is futile or _____ (hopeful, hopeless).

CHAPTER FIFTEEN

NEONATAL MECHANICAL VENTILATION

INTUBATION

1. In addition to an Apgar score of 3 or less obtained immediately after delivery, intubation of a neonate should be considered under all of the following conditions *except*:

   A. ineffective bag/mask ventilation.

   B. presence of thick meconium in the amniotic fluid.

   C. premature rupture of amniotic membrane.

   D. presence of diaphragmatic hernia.

2. Intubation is also indicated in the presence of _____ (obstructive lesions, restrictive defects) such as Pierre-Robin syndrome, tracheomalacia, tracheal web, tracheal stenosis, laryngeal paralysis, and extrinsic masses.

3. Other indications of endotracheal intubation may include all of the following *except*:

   A. removal of secretions.

   B. administration of oxygen.

   C. mechanical ventilation.

   D. collection of tracheal specimens.

4. The Apgar scores range from 0 to _____ and it is usually done immediately after birth (usually called 1-minute Apgar), and after _____ or _____ minutes.

5. Immediately after delivery, a neonate shows the following signs: heart rate of 110/min, irregular and shallow respiratory effort, well flexed muscle tone, grimace upon stimulation, and pink body but blue extremities. The total Apgar score for this assessment is _____ points. What are the individual scores for these five criteria?

   _____

   _____

   _____

6. The laryngoscope blade used in intubation is usually size _____ for most new-borns and all preemies. Some newborns and older infants (generally > 5 kg) require a size _____ .

7 to 9. Match the weights (gestational ages) with the respective ET tube sizes. Use only *four* of the answers provided.

WEIGHT (GESTATIONAL AGE)	TUBE SIZE (mm ID)
7. Below 1000 gm (Below 28 weeks)	A. 1.5
8. 1000 to 2000 gm (28 to 34 weeks)	B. 2.5
9. 2000 to 3000 gm (34 to 38 weeks)	C. 3.0
	D. 3.5
	E. 4.0

10. Each intubation attempt should be limited to less than _____ seconds to minimize hypoxia. It should be stopped sooner if the patient's condition dictates.

11. Describe the method to minimize hypoxia between prolonged intubation attempts.

_____

_____

_____

SURFACTANT REPLACEMENT THERAPY

12. The primary cause of respiratory distress syndrome in the premature neonates is _____ .

13. Surfactant is a naturally occurring substance composed mainly of several _____ (sugars, carbohydrates, lipids, proteins).

14. About 90% of the surfactant is _____, with phosphatidylcholine (PC) comprising 85% of the total amount.

15. About 60% of the PC is dipalmitoyl phosphatidylcholine (DPPC), a substance that allows surfactant to _____ (increase, lower) surface tension.

16. After many years of research, surfactant is found to be most effective when given by _____ (aerosol administration, intravenous administration, direct instillation) into the _____ (lungs, systemic circulation, trachea).

17. _____ (Prophylactic, Therapeutic) administration of surfactant is indicated for those infants who are at a high risk of developing respiratory distress syndrome.

18. Infants who are at risk of developing respiratory distress syndrome are those:
    A. born after 32 weeks of gestation.
    B. with birth weight more than 1300 grams.
    C. with an L/S ratio of 1:1.
    D. with phosphatidylglycerol (PG) in the amniotic fluid.

19. _____ (Prophylactic, Therapeutic) administration of surfactant is not given until the patient develops signs of respiratory distress syndrome.

20. Therapeutic or rescue administration of surfactant is indicated in infants with all of the following signs *except*:

    A. respiratory distress syndrome.

    B. progressive hypoxemia.

    C. ground glass appearance on chest radiograph.

    D. hyperventilation.

21. Respiratory distress syndrome is present when all of the following clinical signs are observed with the *exception* of:

    A. respiratory alkalosis.

    B. grunting.

    C. nasal flaring.

    D. chest retractions.

22. Currently there are two surfactants which are FDA-approved. _____ (Exosurf Neonatal®, Survanta®) is produced by mincing cow lung tissue, whereas _____ (Exosurf Neonatal®, Survanta®) is a synthetic preparation.

23. Surfactant replacement therapy has been used successfully to reduce the severity of _____ (respiratory distress syndrome, cystic fibrosis, meconium aspiration syndrome) and the incidence of some related cardiopulmonary complications.

24. Surfactant replacement therapy _____ (does, does not) work on all patients and it has been implicated in the development of _____ (pulmonary hypertension, intraventricular hemorrhage, interstitial emphysema) in some neonates.

BASIC PRINCIPLES OF NEONATAL VENTILATION

25. Most of the mechanical ventilators used in the neonatal population are classified as pressure-limited ventilators. They deliver variable _____ (pressures, pressure support, tidal volumes, flow) at a preset _____ (pressure, volume, flow, PEEP) limit.

26. The tidal volumes delivered by a pressure-limited ventilator are dependent on the:

    A. patient's compliance.

    B. air flow resistance.

    C. pressure setting.

    D. all of the above.

27. In general, a(n) _____ (increasing, decreasing) compliance or a(n) _____ (increasing, decreasing) airway resistance requires a higher pressure limit to maintain the same tidal volume.

28. When a pressure-limited ventilator is used, the delivered tidal volume _____ (increases, decreases) as the patient's respiratory condition improves. Explain why.

29. The pressure setting on a pressure-limited ventilator should be reduced as the patient's compliance is _____ (increased, decreased) or the airway resistance is _____ (increased, decreased). Explain why.

_____

_____

30. Compressible volume is defined as the portion of ventilator volume that is _____ (added to, lost within) the ventilator circuit and humidifier during the inspiratory phase.

31. To minimize volume loss caused by expansion of the ventilator circuit, the circuit should have a _____ (large, small) compression factor.

32. Neonatal ventilator circuits should have a very _____ (high, low) compression factor so that the patient may receive the largest tidal volume possible from the ventilator.

33. To minimize volume loss within the humidifier, the humidifier used in a neonatal ventilator should also have a _____ (large, small) compressible volume.

34. Condensation or "rain-out" in the ventilator circuit occurs because of the temperature _____ (increase, drop) as the gas goes from the humidifier through the patient circuit.

35. What are three potential problems when the water accumulates in the ventilator tubing?

_____

_____

36. A water trap placed in-line on the _____ (inspiratory, expiratory) side of the ventilator circuit helps to prevent the problems caused by water accumulated in the circuit.

37. Heated wire may be placed inside the _____ (inspiratory, expiratory) tubing to reduce condensation in the ventilator circuit.

38. Premature shut down (power off) of the heated wire may occur if the distal temperature probe is placed at the patient connection _____ (inside, outside) a heated incubator. Explain why.

_____

_____

_____

39. To prevent premature shut down (power off) of the heated wire, the temperature probe should be placed:
    A. outside the inlet to the incubator.
    B. inside the incubator.
    C. at the endotracheal tube adaptor.
    D. inside the expiratory tubing.

INITIATION OF NEONATAL VENTILATOR SUPPORT

40. Indications for neonatal ventilatory support is based on the following general guidelines *except*:

    A. heart rate.

    B. apnea.

    C. hypercapnia.

    D. hypoxemia.

41. A physician wants to increase the tidal volume delivered to the neonate by a pressure-limited ventilator. This is commonly done by:

    A. increasing the pressure limit.

    B. increasing the tidal volume.

    C. decreasing the flow rate.

    D. decreasing the inspiratory time.

42. Which of the following is *not* a primary function of mechanical ventilation?

    A. prevention or correction of atelectasis

    B. oxygenation

    C. removal of carbon dioxide

    D. regulation of metabolic acid-base balance

43. The initial pressure setting on the ventilator should be slightly higher for neonates with _____ (high, low) compliance.

44. For infants with pulmonary air leaks, the initial pressure setting on the ventilator should be slightly _____ (higher, lower) in conjunction with a _____ (faster, slower) mechanical rate.

45 to 51. Complete the *initial* ventilator settings for neonates with normal and low compliance.

PARAMETER	NORMAL COMPLIANCE	LOW COMPLIANCE
45. PIP	_____ to _____ cm H_2O	_____ to _____ cm H_2O
46. PEEP	_____ to _____ cm H_2O	up to _____ cm H_2O
47. V_T	_____ to _____ mL/kg	_____ to _____ mL/kg
48. Rate	_____ /min	Up to _____ /min (esp. with air leak)
49. Flow Rate	_____ to _____ LPM	_____ to _____ LPM
50. I Time	_____ sec	Change according to rate to maintain an I:E ratio of _____
51. I:E Ratio	_____ to _____	At least _____

52. The initial F_IO_2 setting on a neonatal ventilator should be adjusted gradually to keep the patient pink using _____ (SvO_2, SpO_2) or transcutaneous _____ (pH, pCO_2, pO_2) measurements.

53. On a pressure-limited ventilator, the inspiratory time and flow rate are set at 0.5 sec and 7 lpm, respectively. What is the estimated tidal volume?
    A. 14 ml
    B. 35 ml
    C. 58 ml
    D. 140 ml

54. The normal umbilical arterial blood gases for neonates are: PO_2 >_____ mmHg, $PaCO_2$ _____ to _____ mmHg, and pH _____ to _____.

55. For capillary samples, a _____ (higher, lower) PO_2 is expected and considered acceptable.

HIGH FREQUENCY VENTILATION (HFV)

56. High frequency ventilation (HFV) is a technique of ventilation that delivers _____ (large, normal, small) tidal volumes at very high frequencies.

57. How does HFV affect the peak airway pressure and the incidence of barotrauma?

    _____

    _____

58. The use of HFV is often limited to those situations in which _____ (spontaneous ventilation, conventional mechanical ventilation, pressure support ventilation) has failed.

59. HFV appears to be most useful in treating _____ and pneumonia.

60. The rates or frequencies generated by high frequency ventilators are measured in Hertz or cycles/min. One Hertz equals to 1 cycle/*sec* or _____ cycles/*min.*

61. The major types of high frequency ventilator are categorized by the _____ of ventilation and the method with which the _____ is delivered.

62. High frequency positive pressure ventilation (HFPPV) delivers _____ (conventional, jet, pulsating) ventilatory breaths at rates between _____ and _____ breaths per minute.

63. Describe the general indication of high frequency positive pressure ventilation.

    _____

    _____

64. In patients with severely non-compliant lungs, a high respiratory rate may help to _____ (increase, decrease) the peak inspiratory pressure requirement for the delivery of an adequate tidal volume.

65. MAWP = [RR × I time / 60] × (PIP − PEEP) + PEEP

From the equation shown above, the mean airway pressure (MAWP) is _____ (directly, inversely) related to the respiratory rate (RR). Therefore, at high respiratory rate settings, HFPPV tends to _____ (increase, decrease) the MAWP, risk of barotrauma, and cardiac compromise.

66. High frequency jet ventilator (HFJV) delivers a high pressure _____ (tidal volume, pulse of gas) to the patient airway via a special adaptor attached to the endotracheal tube.

67. High frequency jet ventilators (HFJV) operate at rates between _____ and _____ per minute or _____ and _____ Hertz.

68. The indications for using high frequency jet ventilator include severe pulmonary disease that is complicated by all of the following *except*:
    A. pulmonary hypotension.
    B. air leaks.
    C. pulmonary hypoplasia.
    D. restrictive lung disease.

69. High frequency jet ventilation is used:
    A. after conventional ventilation has failed.
    B. to provide intrapulmonary percussion.
    C. in tandem with conventional ventilator.
    D. for premies with respiratory distress syndrome.

70. Which of the following is *not* a purpose of the conventional ventilator when used in tandem with HFJV?
    A. Its sigh breaths stimulate production of surfactant.
    B. Its sigh breaths prevent microatelectasis.
    C. It provides pressure support ventilation.
    D. It provides a continuous gas flow for entrainment by HFJV.

71. What is the major hazard of HFJV due to the impact of high pressure gas on the wall of the airways?

_____

_____

72. To minimize the impact of high pressure gas on the wall of the airways, HFJV should only be delivered through a special catheter that exits _____ (externally, internally) to the endotracheal tube or via a special triple-lumen endotracheal tube.

73. Besides necrotizing tracheobronchitis, name at least three other hazards of HFJV.

_____

_____

74. Why is auscultation of breath sounds and heart sounds difficult during high frequency jet ventilation?

_____

_____

75. In place of auscultation, patient assessment during HFJV may be based on other clinical signs. Decreased lung compliance or pneumothoraces are observed by a(n) _____ (increase, decrease) in chest wall vibration, _____ (hypercapnia, hypocapnia), and _____ (hyperoxia, hypoxemia).

76. During HFJV, a(n) _____ (increase, decrease) in chest wall vibration and a(n) _____ (increase, decrease) in $PaCO_2$, without a drop in PaO_2, may indicate airway obstruction or malposition of the endotracheal tube.

77. Tension pneumothoraces in the neonates may be detected by _____ without using chest radiography.

78. High frequency oscillatory ventilation (HFOV) utilizes the highest of rates, usually in the range of _____ to _____ per minute or _____ to _____ Hertz.

79. A unique feature of the high frequency oscillatory ventilator is that it produces extremely rapid _____ cycles.
    A. inspiratory
    B. expiratory
    C. inspiratory and expiratory
    D. spontaneous breathing

80. Modern high frequency oscillatory ventilators may be provided with simple traditional endotracheal tubes and are not used in tandem with conventional ventilators.

    (TRUE/FALSE)

81. High frequency oscillatory ventilation (HFOV) is indicated for use on neonates with severe _____ complicated with pulmonary _____ (hypertension, hypotension) and _____ (hypercapnia, hypocapnia).

82. High frequency oscillatory ventilation is also effective in stabilizing neonates with congenital _____ (diaphragmatic hernia, heart defects).

83. What is the significance of development of air leaks and failure to show early improvement during HFOV?

    _____

    _____

84. High frequency oscillatory ventilation _____ (enhances, prevents) the release of inflammatory chemical mediators in the lung, resulting in less _____ (cardiovascular complications, lung injuries) than is seen with conventional ventilation.

85. When high frequency oscillatory ventilation is used in conjunction with _____ replacement therapy soon after birth, the incidence and severity of bronchopulmonary dysplasia may be reduced.

86. The ability of HFOV to oxygenate the blood is _____ (better than, equally effective as, not as good as) other methods. Use of _____ (high, low) levels of PEEP is generally done.

87. During HFJV and HFOV, signs of pallor, cyanosis, _____ (tachycardia, bradycardia), _____ (hypertension, hypotension), and increased respiratory effort are indicative of a worsening patient status.

OTHER METHODS OF VENTILATION

88. Perfluorochemicals (PFC) are _____ (gases, liquids, powders) that have been used successfully to support _____ (perfusion, respiration) at very _____ (high, low) pulmonary _____ (blood pressure, inflation pressure).

EXTRACORPOREAL MEMBRANE OXYGENATION (ECMO)

89. Extracorporeal membrane oxygenation (ECMO) is a technique to oxygenate the blood _____ (by a ventilator, by blood transfusion, outside the body).

90. ECMO is not recommended for infants of less than _____ weeks of gestational age, weighing less than _____ grams, having evidence of _____ hemorrhage.

91. ECMO is contraindicated when mechanical ventilation has been used for more than _____ weeks prior to the initiation of ECMO. This is because of an increased incidence of _____ (pulmonary hypertension, congestive heart failure, chronic lung disease), which ECMO cannot reverse.

92. Potential candidates for ECMO may include those with congenital heart defects since ECMO does not interfere with ventilation.

    (TRUE/FALSE)

93. ECMO therapy is reserved for candidates with extremely high mortality rate (80% or greater) under conventional mechanical ventilation strategies. Which of the following methods is not used to predict mortality?
    A. Alveolar-arterial oxygen pressure gradient [$P(A-a)O_2$]
    B. Oxygen index
    C. Oxygen consumption and cardiac output
    D. PaO_2 or pH measurements

94. A $P(A-a)O_2$ value of _____ to _____ mm Hg at 100% F_IO_2 for 4 to 12 hours is indicative for ECMO therapy since it is consistent with _____ (mild, moderate, severe) hypoxemia.

95. A neonate has the following umbilical arterial blood gases: pH = 7.34, $PaCO_2$ = 45 mm Hg, PaO_2 = 68 mm Hg, F_IO_2 = 100%. What is the $P(A-a)O_2$ if the barometric pressure is 748 mm Hg?
    A. 588 mm Hg
    B. 635 mm Hg
    C. 680 mm Hg
    D. 703 mm Hg

96. Infants with an oxygen index of _____ to _____ for 0.5 to 6 hours are inclusive for ECMO therapy because this condition reflects _____ (high, low) airway pressures in conjunction with hypoxemia.

97. An infant has the following measurements: mean airway pressure = 25 cm H_2O, PaO_2 = 45 mm Hg at an F_IO_2 of 60%. What is the calculated oxygen index?

    A. 15

    B. 33

    C. 67

    D. 82

98. A third criteria for ECMO therapy is the presence of a PaO_2 of _____ to _____ mm Hg for 2 to 12 hours or a pH of less than _____ for 2 hours with _____ (hypertension, hypotension).

99. In the venoarterial route, blood is drawn from the _____ (left, right) atrium via the _____ (external, internal) jugular vein. The oxygenated blood is returned to the _____ via the right common _____ (brachial, femoral, carotid) artery.

100. Explain how the venoarterial ECMO supports the cardiac function of the patient.

    _____

    _____

101. In the venovenous route, blood is removed from the _____ (left, right) atrium via the _____ (left, right) internal jugular vein. The oxygenated blood is returned to the _____ (aortic arch, right atrium, left atrium) through a catheter inserted via the _____ vein.

102. The venovenous method oxygenates the blood and it also supports a patient's cardiac output.

    (TRUE/FALSE)

103. List at least three *pulmonary* complications of ECMO.

    _____

    _____

104. What are the two major *cardiovascular* complications of ECMO?

    _____

    _____

105. _____ (Polycythemia, Anemia), _____ (leukocytosis, leukopenia) and _____ (thrombocytosis, thrombocytopenia) are possible hematologic complications of ECMO. This is caused by the _____ (creation, consumption) of blood components by the membrane oxygenator.

CHAPTER SIXTEEN

HOME MECHANICAL VENTILATION

GOALS OF HOME VENTILATOR CARE

1. There are several advantages to be gained by providing mechanical ventilation in the patient's home. They include all of the following *except*:

   A. extension and enhancement of quality of life.

   B. improvement of patient's physical and physiological functions.

   C. reduction of cost for mechanical ventilation.

   D. reduction of stress level of family members.

2. At home, the patient on mechanical ventilation is more likely to become _____ (more active, indifferent, more passive) in the weaning or rehabilitation process.

3. Interactions with family members and friends at home will enhance the patient's _____ (physical, spiritual, psychological, medical) well being and quality of life.

4. Since the cost savings of providing mechanical ventilation at home can be drastic, it should be the primary consideration in sending a patient from the hospital to home.

   (TRUE/FALSE)

5. The most important ingredient of a successful home ventilator care program is probably the:

   A. financial resources of the patient.

   B. dedication and commitment of home care team members.

   C. insurance policy of the patient.

   D. availability of state-of-the-art equipment.

INDICATIONS

6. What are the four questions that may be helpful in assessing the indications for providing mechanical ventilation at home?

_____

_____

_____

_____

_____

_____

_____

_____

7 to 10. Many different diseases may be managed with home mechanical ventilation. Match the pulmonary problems with the respective clinical courses. Use each answer only once.

PULMONARY PROBLEM CLINICAL COURSE

7. COPD
8. Restrictive Lung Disease
9. Ventilatory Muscle Dysfunction
10. Central Hypoventilation Syndrome

A. Inefficient ventilatory muscle → Atelectasis → pneumonia

B. Apnea → Chronic hypoventilation → Atelectasis → pneumonia

C. Reduction of lung volumes and capacities → Dead space ventilation → Muscle fatigue

D. Air flow obstruction → Excessively high compliance → Air trapping → Acute exacerbation

11. Patients with stable Chronic Obstructive Pulmonary Disease (COPD) typically have blood gases showing _____ (acute, chronic) ventilatory failure or _____ (compensated, uncompensated) respiratory acidosis.

12. When COPD patients develop ventilatory failure or oxygenation failure, blood gases usually show _____ (acute, chronic) ventilatory failure superimposed on _____ (acute, chronic) ventilatory failure.

13. Define acute exacerbation of COPD.

_____

_____

_____

14. Which of the following blood gas reports best illustrates acute exacerbation of COPD?

    A. pH = 7.36, $PaCO_2$ = 55 mm Hg, PaO_2 = 50 mm Hg, HCO_3^- = 30 mEq/L

    B. pH = 7.38, $PaCO_2$ = 46 mm Hg, PaO_2 = 75 mm Hg, HCO_3^- = 26 mEq/L

    C. pH = 7.27, $PaCO_2$ = 74 mm Hg, PaO_2 = 43 mm Hg, HCO_3^- = 33 mEq/L

    D. pH = 7.20, $PaCO_2$ = 42 mm Hg, PaO_2 = 43 mm Hg, HCO_3^- = 16 mEq/L

15. Why are COPD patients more difficult to wean off mechanical ventilation?

    _____

    _____

16. The primary problem of restrictive lung disease is the reduction of _____ (air flow, lung volumes). Patients with restrictive lung disease usually assume a _____ (rapid and shallow, slow and deep) breathing pattern.

17. The amount of dead space ventilation is _____ (increased, decreased) in rapid shallow breathing because the anatomic dead space volume is _____ (increased, stable, decreased) with this breathing pattern.

18. The work of breathing in restrictive lung diseases is _____ (higher, lower) than normal because of the _____ (high, low) lung compliance characteristic.

19. Patients with uncomplicated ventilatory muscle dysfunction usually have _____ (healthy, unhealthy) lungs.

20. Under what conditions do restrictive lung patients need mechanical ventilation?

    _____

    _____

    _____

21. A patient who was in a fall accident sustained high spinal cord injuries at the cervical 2 (C-2) level. This patient is most likely a candidate for long-term:

    A. aerosol therapy.

    B. nasal CPAP therapy.

    C. BiPAP therapy.

    D. mechanical ventilation.

22. Regardless of the etiology, patients with central hypoventilation syndrome often require around-the-clock mechanical ventilation.

    (TRUE/FALSE)

23. What are the primary pulmonary problems of persistent hypoventilation due to dysfunction of the autonomic control of breathing?

    _____

    _____

PATIENT SELECTION

24. What are the two criteria that preclude a hospitalized patient from receiving mechanical ventilation at home?

_____

_____

25. In addition to the medical criteria that are used for home care discharge planning, the decision should also be based on the desires of the:
    A. physician.
    B. patient.
    C. insurance carrier.
    D. hospital administrator.

26. Potential candidates for home ventilator care should be told about the potential _____ (advantages, disadvantages, advantages and disadvantages) of leaving the hospital and entering a home care environment.

27. List two *advantages* gained by a ventilator-dependent patient leaving the hospital and entering a home care environment.

_____

_____

28. List two *disadvantages* experienced by a ventilator-dependent patient leaving the hospital and entering a home care environment.

_____

_____

29. Explain why the discussions concerning home ventilator care should not take place when the patient is hypoxic, confused, or under emotional distress.

_____

_____

30. Why is it essential that the desires of the family members be considered before making plans for home mechanical ventilation?

_____

_____

31. What are the two major expenses of home ventilator care?

_____

32. Home ventilator care can be justified from a financial standpoint when its total cost is _____ (higher than, same as, lower than) the cost of comparable hospital care.

33. Adequate space for the ventilator, special bed, wheelchair, oxygen units, and supplies are some concerns that deal with the _____ (physical environment, technical support, emotional support) provided for the patient receiving home ventilator care.

EQUIPMENT SELECTION

34. If the patient does not have adequate spontaneous ventilation for an extended time, _____ are the equipment of choice.
    A. chest cuirass and pneumobelt
    B. raincoat and wrap
    C. rocking bed and diaphragmatic pacing
    D. positive pressure or negative pressure ventilators

35. Under what condition is a backup ventilator necessary in a home care setting?

    _____

    _____

36. One negative-pressure ventilation device that resembles a shell fitting over the patient's chest wall is called a _____ (chest cuirass, raincoat or wrap, pneumobelt, rocking bed).

37. The _____ is another negative-pressure ventilation device that is an airtight jacket capable of sealing the arms, hips, and neck.

38. Explain how the pneumobelt provides ventilation.

    _____

    _____

39. The rocking bed relies on _____ (positive pressure, negative pressure, motion) to displace the abdominal contents to facilitate diaphragmatic motion and ventilation.

40. Diaphragmatic pacing _____ (provides, augments) ventilation by stimulation of the thoracic _____ (arteries, veins, phernic nerves).

41. Why should a home care ventilator be extremely dependable?

    _____

    _____

42. Why should a home care ventilator be simple to operate?

    _____

    _____

43. What are two advantages of ventilators with built-in rechargable battery packs?

    _____

    _____

LEARNING OBJECTIVES FOR POSITIVE PRESSURE VENTILATION IN THE HOME

44. The learning objectives for positive pressure ventilation in the home can be a very useful resource for all of the following personnel *except*:

    A. family members.

    B. respiratory and nursing care personnel.

    C. discharge planners.

    D. health care policymakers.

45. The learning objectives for positive pressure ventilation in the home should be used in its entirety for each patient receiving home ventilator care.

    (TRUE/FALSE)

46. Who should be responsible for selecting and modifying the learning objectives prior to initiation of home ventilator care?

    _____

    _____

47. Once the learning objectives are _____ (read, discussed, met), the patient and caregivers may begin to use the ventilator independently at home, initially under supervision and guidance.

48. Why should the learning objectives be accompanied by other specific information and materials on equipment, supplies, or procedure?

    _____

    _____